ON CALL

ON CALL

A Doctor's Days and Nights in Residency

Emily R. Transue, M.D.

St. Martin's Griffin ♏ New York

www.stmartins.com

Design by Jane Adele Regina

Library of Congress Cataloging-in-Publication Data

Transue, Emily R.
    On call : a doctor's days and nights in residency / Emily R. Transue.
        p. cm.
    ISBN 0-312-32483-9 (hc)
    ISBN 0-312-32484-7 (pbk)
    EAN 978-0-312-32484-1
    1. Transue, Emily R. 2. Interns (Medicine)—United States—Biography.
3. Physician and patient. I. Title.

R154.T673 A3 2004
610'.92—dc22   2004046893
[B]

First St. Martin's Griffin Edition: August 2005

10 9 8 7 6 5 4 3 2 1

To Harriet F. Adams, J.D., Ph.D.

My mother, teacher, inspiration, friend

Note to Readers

The names and identifying characteristics of all patients have been changed to preserve confidentiality. Names of physicians and staff have also been changed to protect their anonymity.

Contents

Acknowledgments

I would like to acknowledge the following, without whom this book would never have come into existence: Chris Pepin, who made residency bearable—here's to never having to do it again. Blair Brooks, who started all this by reading an e-mail—I promise I'll read aloud more slowly this time around. My wonderful agent, Joan Raines, and her partner, Theron Raines, for believing in me and in the book. Diane Reverand, Gina Scarpa, and everyone at St. Martin's Press. Roxanne Young at JAMA, for crucial early support and encouragement. Dana Grossman and the staff of *Dartmouth Medicine*, fabulous people and staunch supporters of my writing all along—they first published several of these stories, and were most generous in releasing Web rights. Doug Paauw, Erika Goldstein, Chris Surawicz, and Connie Celum, who have continued to nurture both my literary and my medical career. Alison Samitt, Shala Erlich, Dennis Rivet, and Ellen Gerety, wonderful readers as well as friends. Kit Transue, John Straub, and William and Monique Transue, the most supportive family anyone could have. My father, Jacques Transue, who will always be part of everything I do; he would have been proud to see this published. Chris Knight, for nursing me through the birth pains of this book, doing everything from copyediting to technical support to reassembling the despairing author whenever she fell apart. Most of all, my patients, for teaching me and sharing their stories with me. This is their book.

ON CALL

Prologue

It was a misty New Hampshire morning, July 1994. The silence was broken by a siren, an ambulance racing toward the pretty white-and-green hospital in the woods. I was a medical student in my first week of clinical work. I helped wheel the woman on the stretcher out of the ambulance and into Emergency. I watched as her clothes were cut off and replaced with tubes and monitors. I helped pound on her chest until at last she was declared dead.

How does a person react to an event like this? I had woken up that morning having never seen a death, and by lunchtime I had been part of one. Nothing in medical school or in life had prepared me for that moment. Amid the jumble of predictable emotions—sadness, fear, confusion, a certain excitement—I felt wrenchingly and terribly alone. I had seen a heart stop, I had felt ribs break under my thrusting palms. The people I loved best in the world were not in medicine. Would they understand what I had just seen and done? Would I be inevitably separated from them by this experience and those that would follow it?

I did the only thing I could think of. I sat down that afternoon and wrote it all down. If I could tell my mother, my brother, my friend in film school, exactly what had happened, then I wouldn't be alone. And maybe, while trying to make them understand, I would come to understand it, too.

That first story, sent out as an e-mail, led to more stories. What began as a way of staying connected to my loved ones outside medicine became a way of staying connected to myself. Writing became a part of the practice of medicine for me, a guard against numbness and burnout, a reminder to listen closely to each patient and to my feelings as I interacted with them. As I shared the stories, first with friends and later through publication, I discovered that my experiences, which often felt so solitary and isolating, resonated with those of other students and doctors. I was shy at first in confessing to my patients that I wrote, though I tried to ask permission when I wrote their stories down. To my surprise, patients and their families said the stories gave them a better sense of the "other side" of medicine.

I graduated from medical school in 1996, and moved to Seattle to begin my residency—postgraduate specialty training—in Internal Medicine. I was twenty-four, a few years younger than most of my colleagues, having graduated from college at twenty and gone straight through to medical school. I would become an internist, a "pediatrician for adults," responsible for all aspects of adult care except surgery and obstetrics. My residency training would last three years, of which the first, the internship year, would be the most exhausting and intense. In Seattle's program, I would rotate among four hospitals: the university hospital, specializing in the more obscure problems, the county hospital, the center for trauma and indigent care, the Veteran's Administration or VA hospital, and a private community hospital. I would rotate among months in the Intensive Care Unit, on the general medical wards or "ward services," in such specialties as Cardiology and Oncology, and in the Emergency Room. In general, I would spend every fourth night "on call," spending the night in the hospital as well as the day before and after. I would get four days off each month. For half a day each week during the three years, I would have my own clinic, a "continuity clinic" where I would be a primary care doctor for a group of patients. I would also have "clinic blocks," months spent in my continuity clinic and in a variety of specialty clinics, with no weekend work or call.

By the time I started internship, medicine and writing were entwined for me. As things happened I wrote them down, scribbling fragments of conversation on the backs of my patient notecards. Sometimes I would weave these fragments into stories right away, sometimes I waited months or years. In the most exhausting times, all I could do was keep a few barely intelligible notes. But even these reminded me to stay in the moment, to cherish my experiences, the hard as well as the happy ones, the shameful as well as the proud.

This book is a compilation of those experiences, beginning on the first morning of my residency and ending on its final night. I have tried to capture some of what I learned in those long and difficult years. Names and other details have been changed to protect confidentiality, but otherwise I have tried to render both the people and the medicine accurately.

If I had to describe my experience of becoming a physician in two words, one would be "fatigue." The mental, physical, and emotional exhaustion of this process is a theme that runs throughout this book. The other would be "gratitude." These difficult, dark years were brightened at every point by the friends and colleagues who taught me and learned with me. The medical training system can be brutal in some ways, but the people within it are deeply supportive of each other. I am honored to have such friends. Most of all, I am grateful to my patients and their families. I learned more from them than from anyone—medical lessons as well as life lessons. The great joy and privilege of medicine is being welcomed into people's lives in critical and quiet moments, being invited to share their stories. It is these stories that make up this book.

1. A Long White Coat

Medicine is a secret society of sorts, a world unto itself, with its own language, codes, and symbols. One of the subtle but powerful codes is found in the hierarchy of the white coats. Medical students wear short coats, to the waist or hip. Interns and residents—recent graduates in their first and subsequent years of specialty training—wear long coats, knee-length, grown-up coats. Beyond that the distinctions are more subtle; attendings—teaching doctors, who have finished training—wear classier coats, with braided cloth buttons. But the primary difference is in the length: when you become a doctor, you wear a long white coat.

For me, this was the strongest symbol of the passage into internship. More than the pomp and circumstance of graduation, with all of its glorious moments: turning to face the assembled crowd as my mentor laid a green stole around my neck, whispering in my ear, "Now you're official—"; the reciting of the Hippocratic oath; the proclamation of the dean and president, "I hereby bestow upon you the degree of Doctor of Medicine. . . ." More than the heart-wrenching good-byes to my medical school friends, the abrupt and painful dismantling of my apartment, packing all my possessions into a truck and driving three thousand miles across the nation. More than any of those things, what made me suddenly realize I'd become a doctor was looking into a mirror on my first morning of work at the county hospital in Seattle and seeing my reflection in a long white coat.

Probably it's a result of years of conditioning and constant reinforcement: people in short coats are students, long ones are doctors. There are places that don't use this system, a few hospitals in the country where interns, or all residents, wear short coats. But it's bred into me now: the long coat is synonymous with authority, with competence. The coat seems stronger than my own persona, I try to become the person who is wearing it. I notice myself adjusting my posture, my bearing, to match the coat. I occasionally allowed myself a certain frivolity as a student, which seems inappropriate in this new attire. Act your age, the coat seems to insist. You are a doctor now.

MY FIRST MORNING of internship, I plan to get to the hospital an hour early, have breakfast in the cafeteria, arrive at clinic calm and settled. But the morning is fraught with delays, as I struggle to find my stethoscope, not seen since the move, I suddenly realize, my name tag, which was in one of the two dozen envelopes I've been given in the last two days, my parking pass, in yet another envelope, my pager. I get lost on the way to the hospital, then realize I have no idea where I'm supposed to park. I arrive with just enough time to find my clinic. Five South, my schedule says. I take the center elevators, the only ones I know, to the fifth floor, step out into a corridor of small doors with prominent locks and tiny windows. In fact, I realize as the elevator doors close behind me, 5 Center is a locked psychiatric ward. There is no door to 5 South, there's no reentry to the elevator without a key, there are no staff in sight.

At the moment I become, officially, an intern—my first moment as a real doctor—I am involuntarily locked on a psychiatric ward. Despite my near tears of panic and frustration, I have to laugh at the image: I could imagine getting committed at some point in this whole residency process, but I didn't envision it happening quite this early. . . .

I wander around and finally find a nurse. "I'm a new intern," I say. "I was looking for Five South, and I accidentally got here. . . ."

I imagine her saying, "Sure you did. Go back to your room. Where'd you get that coat?" Instead, she just giggles and reaches for her elevator key.

Later I'll learn there is a term for this: *July*. July is when the new interns come, eager and foolish and amusing to everyone else.

* * *

My FIRST MORNING is Geriatrics clinic, in a clinic wing of the hospital building. Although I'm a little late from my detour to the psych ward, the attending physician hasn't arrived yet. I set down my bag, and start to introduce myself to the senior resident in the staff room. "Hi," I say, the force of habit taking over. "I'm Emily Transue, I'm a med stu—"

And then I stop, stricken. She looks at me, smiles an ever-so-slight knowing smile, and says: "No, you're not."

A few minutes later, in walks an actual medical student. I introduce myself, noting his short coat. "You're a student?"

"Third year," he says, smiling weakly. "Very new . . ."

He looks so young—

I think of myself as being him, I realize suddenly. But I'm not.

The attending—the senior doctor in clinic for the day—arrives, shows me around the clinic, explains some procedural things. Then he leads me to the exam room where my first patient is waiting.

"This is Dr. Transue," he tells the patient. "She's one of our interns. She'll be seeing you today and helping you with your issues. I'll be in later as well, to confirm what the two of you decide."

This is Dr. Transue. I stare dumbly at the attending for a moment, mesmerized by his words. I've waited for this for so long, worked for it for so many years. But now that it's happening, I'm not sure whether to be thrilled or terrified.

He smiles at both of us, then steps out of the room, closing the door behind him. I turn to the patient, who is watching me expectantly.

"Hi," I say, smiling and shaking her hand. I gesture to her to have a seat on the exam table. I sit down in the swivel chair at the room's small desk, lay down her chart. My heart pounds and my mouth is dry. I reach for the familiar phrases and motions of this role for which I have spent so many years preparing.

"Tell me what brings you here today."

2. Hepatoma

Clinic block, with which I began my residency, is a mélange of things: a variety of teaching conferences on common outpatient medical problems, time spent in subspecialty clinics like Pulmonary and Cardiology. The heart of it lies in "continuity clinic," my own general medicine clinic. I'll spend a half day per week here through the three years of residency, even when I'm working on the hospital wards. I have a "panel" of a few hundred patients inherited from a graduating resident, to which I'll add more over time, who are my own set of patients, those for whom I will be the primary care doctor. I discuss them with the clinic attendings, and I can refer them to subspecialists, but I am their doctor. It is thrilling yet daunting to step into this role and realize that there are a group of people—people out there living their lives—who belong to you, who are your responsibility.

I ARRIVE ON my first day of continuity clinic, my first day of meeting these patients who are so uniquely mine. The attending in charge shows me around, pointing out my room, the lab, the nurses' room, the med closet. He introduces me to the charting system and the lab computer.

"Here's your first chart." He hands me a yellow tome, thick and heavy and impressive. My stomach lurches. Couldn't my first patient have been someone simple and reasonably healthy?

I open the chart, begin to flip through it, adjusting to the new order and format, wondering why every hospital on earth has to have a slightly different charting system. The patient's list of problems is daunting: drug abuse and hepatitis and herpes and alcoholism and a history of pancreatitis and gall bladder disease and chronic low back pain. . . . How am I going to get all this straight, where am I going to start?

I continue through the chart, and suddenly come across something new. Six months ago he had an attack of pain, thought to be gallstones, and an ultrasound showed a mass in his liver. The CT scan, done next, showed a cluster of lesions, felt by the radiologists to be suspicious for hepatoma—hepatocellular carcinoma, cancer of the liver.

The attending, reading over my shoulder, glances at the calendar. "When was this? Six months ago? Probably wasn't a hepatoma then." It's an aggressive and, if not caught very early, untreatable kind of cancer; most people with hepatomas are dead at six months.

I turn the page and find the pathology report: multiple large foci of poorly differentiated hepatocellular carcinoma. From those dry pathology terms it's clear: he's going to die.

You CAN ALMOST hear the crash as my medical armamentarium smashes to the ground. I have been weaving a web as I read the chart, constructing a plan with the information it contains. I am building a framework for how the interview will go, more or less what my plan will be, which issues will be easy or hard to manage, what to work toward in the long run. All of that collapses, now; there is no long run. All of my plans have become suddenly unimportant.

Even though I have been taught, and I believe, that the role of a doctor goes far beyond simple biomedical diagnosis and cure, even though I know that internists rarely solve but often manage problems, and that as much of therapy is in words as in medications, still I am dumbfounded at the simple finality of an untreatable, rapidly fatal disease. He is going to die. There is nothing I can do to change that. I have nothing to offer this man—nothing but pain medication and whatever powers of comfort I may possess.

I feel naked, stripped of my arsenal of now irrelevant technical knowledge and technological power, left with nothing but my small untrained and insufficient self. All that I can do for him is be there for him as he dies. Do I know how to do that? Am I strong enough to do that? To choose to empathize, to care, to believe in a cause that is already lost?

At the same time that his diagnosis fills me with a sense of helplessness and futility, it also carries an overwhelming responsibility. Not only am I now this person's doctor but I am going to be his doctor for the rest of his life. This man is going to die on my watch.

What does it mean, to step into a situation like this one? I've never had to do anything like this before. I envision what will happen. I'll see him every week or two for the few months that this goes on, agonizing over pain meds, how to keep his pain controlled without habituating him to a point at which the medications cease to work. I'll see him pass through stages of coming to terms with his diagnosis and impending death, watch denial and despair. I'll get the call when a crisis brings him to the hospital, in the end; I'll go to see him, even though my medical duties will be discharged then, he'll be in other hands.

There will be more, too, that I don't even think to imagine then. Being my first patient would be only the beginning of a series of firsts he would bring to my young doctoring life. He would be the object of my first (and second, and third and fourth) paracentesis, the draining of fluid from the abdomen, where it builds up behind the failing liver. The two of us would learn together to be experts on the process. He'd sit and I'd stand for hours with my needle in his belly, draining liters of thick yellow ascitic fluid which we would joke looked just like beer, a thick sweet lager. Sometimes we'd chat about his dog or other things, sometimes lapse into the silence of our own respective thoughts, or he would nap while I held the needle in place.

On days I wasn't in clinic, I would check in with him by telephone. I would feel hurt and drained and scared, but he would teach me some strangely positive emotions also: the warmth in the pit of my stomach at being called by his mother to say he was doing a little better and they were headed to the beach for the weekend; the experience of giving them my pager number and feeling not fear at placing myself on call for whatever off-hours problem he might have but relief at knowing I'd be the first to hear about it. And then, at last, I would learn the awful, sick, empty feeling of a death that signified the loss of a friend and that, in spite of everything, felt like my fault. I would be away on a rare week of vacation when he died; I wouldn't be there.

"THAT'S A TOUGH case, to have as your first patient." The gentle voice of the attending breaks into my reverie. I look up into his thoughtful face and concerned eyes, and realize that for him at this moment the patient is not a forty-three-year-old man dying from hepatic cancer but a twenty-four-year-old newly minted doctor embarking on her own strange and difficult journey. Not for the first time it occurs to me how similar doctoring and teaching are. I smile, deeply reassured at the reminder that this is allowed to be hard for me.

I FINISH MY review of the chart. Taking a deep breath, I walk into the room where the patient is seated, waiting.

"Hi," I say.

"Hi," he says.

I look at him carefully. He looks older than his real age, his hair and beard graying, his forehead creased and wrinkled. His belly is distended with fluid, his calves swollen. Yet his eyes and his manner are young—childlike, unsettled, and uncertain.

I introduce myself, explain that I will be taking over from his old doctor, a resident who's just graduated.

He nods.

I ask him how he is.

"Okay, I guess," he says.

What do either of us mean by this question and answer? I don't know.

He tells me about his ascites, the fluid building up in his belly as his liver fails. He says he was just in the hospital, where they took seventeen liters of fluid out of his belly over a couple of days. The hole where they put in the needle for the paracentesis is still draining. In fact, he says, sheepishly, he's leaking through his dressing into his shirt, do we have more gauze?

I don't know where to find anything, so we search together through the drawers for a few awkward moments to find the materials to redress him.

"How has your pain been?" I ask. I'd seen in his chart that he was on very high doses of narcotics.

"The medications help," he says. "I can still feel it—a deep, intense pain in here"—he points to his liver—"but the pills keep it at bay."

I ask about alcohol. He shakes his head quickly. "I quit the day I found out I had the cancer. November nineteenth. Crack, too, and all that other stuff—I'm through with all of it." He shakes his head again, pensively.

"I quit smoking," he adds a little shyly. "That was later, just a couple weeks ago. . . . It was tough, that. Tougher than alcohol almost."

His voice is embarrassed and eager and proud, and I am wounded by his hopefulness. Too little, too late, I think. Even so much. What good does it do you, I want to ask, to give up smoking now? Emphysema and lung cancer and cardiac disease are plagues you have been freed from by more pressing concerns. Part of me wants to say, Go, drink up a storm, smoke like a chimney, have your last laugh and enjoy your last months as best you can.

Instead I am silent, because he will surely get more out of his remaining life this way, clean and clearheaded and pensive.

Yet there are warning bells going off: it's not as simple as that. He's bargaining, I think. He's thinking: If I'm good enough now, maybe it will all go away. One of these days he'll realize that it isn't helping, and then this angelic aura will be transformed into bitterness, because, having been good, it will be no longer his fault, it will be God who rescinded on his half of the bargain. . . .

I don't want to be there for the bitterness. To have him go out drugged and dulled would be easier for me.

"What do you do with your time?" I ask.

"Not much," he says, frowning. "I can't work anymore, I'm not strong enough. I sit around the house a lot. Drive my parents crazy. And a lot of the time I just walk around in the woods with my dog. . . .

"I was always kind of a loner—but now? The people I used to hang out with disgust me. Bunch of winos and junkies. There's no one I want to see really. Just my dog . . ."

He lapses into silence.

"How are your spirits?" I ask gently. I know he's taking antidepressants.

"As good as you could expect them to be, I guess," he says, squinting.

I nod, wait for him to go on.

"Not to say I don't have my moments," he says.

"Tell me about the moments."

"I don't know," he says, after a pause. "I just wonder—what's the point, you know?"

I sigh.

"Sometimes I think I should just go up on a hillside with my dog and shoot the both of us."

I nod slowly.

"I don't think I'll do it, though," he says.

I wait to see what he'll say next.

"Not to say I haven't been up there, in the woods with the gun—"

"What stops you?" I ask, when he doesn't go on.

"My dog, mostly," he says. "I couldn't shoot her. She's all that matters to me."

"How long have you had her?" I ask, because his eyes say he doesn't want to talk more about the depression now.

"Oh, six, eight years now."

"What kind is she?"

"I don't know. Part Lab, I think, part golden. She's not anything exactly, just a mutt I guess. I didn't get her anywhere, just picked her up. She was just a mangy little thing. They were shooting at her, outside a bar. I took her home. . . .

"I didn't really even want a dog," he says. "But there she was. Who'd have known I'd have her longer than anything; my job, my marriage, even—"

Longer than your life, I think.

"It sounds like she means an awful lot to you," I say.

"She's the best friend I have," he says. "You can hit her, and she don't hit back. Not like my wife—"

There's a pause.

"Ex-wife," he adds, under his breath.

Then, glancing up at me, "Sorry—"

I shake my head and even, very wryly, half smile. What am I supposed to say to something like that? Does it matter now? Shall I forgive you all your sins because you are dying? Have I become not a doctor but a priest?

"DID YOU BOND?" The attending smiles kindly at me as I walk back into the residents' room.

"We did, kind of, actually—" Of course, it occurs to me, by bonding I am only letting myself in for an awful heartache.

I present the depression tale, along with the other issues, to my attending, who sighs, looks at me thoughtfully. "Of course—how would you feel if you were dying of liver cancer? If he were, even, to go out into the woods and blow his brains out—would that be unreasonable?"

"Illegal," he adds wryly, "certainly. But unreasonable?..." He sighs. "I don't know."

"I don't know if anyone has discussed end-of-life issues with him," I say. "Code status, hospice questions. I couldn't find it in the chart."

"Then it's probably not there," he says. "Good thought—kind of a rough thing to bring up the first time you see someone, though, isn't it?"

"Yeah," I say heavily.

"If you want, you could wait; you'll be seeing him often, every couple of weeks probably. Wait till you know him a little better, and it will be easier."

I GO BACK in to my patient, and we talk a little more, wrapping up. I write prescriptions for his pain medications and sundry other things—a stool softener for the constipation he gets with the narcotics, and so on—feeling, again, terribly powerless. I make an appointment for him to come back in two weeks. "You're booked," says the secretary. How can I be booked when I only just got here? "Then overbook me," I say, the words giving me a thrill that is half excitement and half terror. I shake his hand and give him my card and my voice-mail number. "If anything comes up, you can call me. Anytime." He nods and walks, shuffling a little from his swollen belly, to the door.

I set down his chart in the resident's room, put off his paperwork until later. I already have two patients waiting.

3. A Partnership

Mr. R appeared in Pulmonary clinic carrying an X-ray and a sheaf of referral slips. He had been applying for a job and had a PPD placed, a skin test for tuberculosis. It was positive, which was not a surprise; he was a native of Thailand and had been exposed as a child. His employer sent him to the TB clinic, where the next step was a chest X-ray, to rule out active disease. The study didn't show tuberculosis; but it was very abnormal, a diffuse, nodular scarring pattern. The TB clinic referred him to Pulmonary, and here he was.

He explains all this to me when I go in to see him. As a new intern on my clinic block, I spend a half day a week in Pulmonary clinic. After he explains why he's here, I ask about his lungs, his breathing.

"I work at the airport," he says. "In the loading section. I lift things off a conveyor belt at the top of a ramp; fumes blow out of the ramp, and they make my eyes water and my mouth burn. I try not to breathe them, but there's no way not to—that's what's wrong with my lungs. I told them, over and over, I make complaints—but they never listen. They don't care."

He sighs. Then adds: "It wasn't the job I wanted. I wanted a job working with people, but they turned me down. They said I couldn't be understood. Because of my accent." He has a thick Thai accent. I have to concentrate to understand his words. "But all the time, people come through the airport, foreigners often, and they're lost, and they ask me where to go. And I tell them, and they understand. It's just a question of wanting to. People can understand if they stop to listen."

I nod. I hear the statement behind his words, too: if I listen, I will understand him, also.

After we've talked—not just about TB, but the rest of his medical situation and history, his life and habits—I leave him, go back to present to the Pulmonary attending. I tell his story, stand at the attending's shoulder as he peers, engrossed, at the X-ray.

"Fascinating," he murmurs. "Just fascinating."

He looks up at me. "What do you think of when you see a noduloreticular pattern?"

You want an honest answer? I think to myself. *When I see a noduloreticular pattern on chest X-ray, I think: nothing.* I know we learned about this in med school, but my mind is drawing a complete blank. Worse, I'm panicking, thinking: *What am I doing here? How am I supposed to succeed as an intern if I can't even remember the differential diagnosis of a noduloreticular chest X-ray?*

Instead of saying this, I merely frown up at him thoughtfully, and eventually he begins listing a differential diagnosis: Idiopathic pulmonary fibrosis. Miliary TB. Sarcoidosis. Asbestosis. Aspergillosis.

I tell him about the fumes at the airport, and he shakes his head dismissively. "Some kind of irritant. This is a different kind of process—maybe an exposure from a long time ago. Did he ever work in bird farming?"

"I don't know," I say.

He looks back up at the X-ray. "Fascinating," he murmurs one more time.

The pulmonologist returns to the examining room with me. He's a tall, kindly man and he talks at length and earnestly in seven-syllable words that obviously mean nothing to the patient. After several minutes, he finishes: "We're going to run a bunch of tests and see you back in a month, okay?"—and the patient manages to get a word in.

"Doctor, I breathe these fumes at work, they make me choke—"

The attending nods, breaks in. "I know. Dr. Transue told me. But that's not what's wrong. Don't worry about that."

He smiles brightly, stands up, reaches for the door.

The patient pauses, then after a moment tries another tack.

"Doctor, I want to stop smoking. I've tried on my own, and I can't. I'm asking you for help—"

"Stopping smoking is a great idea. I'd really encourage that."

He raises an eyebrow at me. "You can write him a prescription for a nicotine patch."

He nods at the patient, shakes his hand in a friendly way, and we leave.

I walk at his side to the staff room feeling a burning sense of things not being right. This has been, in the typical understatement of medical parlance, an "unsatisfying encounter." This is just not working, I think to myself.

Seeking a more positive approach, I try to analyze what's going wrong. He needs someone to sit down and talk with him about what's going on, to deal with him, not just his lungs. He's more complicated than an interesting pulmonary process.

In short, I suddenly realize, this guy needs a primary care doctor. How do I get him a primary care doctor?

I *am* a primary care doctor.

I GO BACK in. "You said Fridays were the one day that was good for you to come in, right?" I say. We'd discussed this earlier—how he works every weekday except Friday, and he's terrified to miss work for fear of losing his job. He may hate it, but he needs it. In fact, he's late today already; he's been anxiously glancing at his watch since halfway through our interview. "Friday is the one day I could really come in and talk," he'd said.

"I want you to come to my continuity clinic on Friday afternoon," I say. "We'll talk about your smoking, and anything else you want to discuss. Okay?"

"Okay," he says.

I walk with him to the front desk to make the appointment. He's about to be late for work by now; there's a lot of paperwork to be done, and the secretary spends several minutes typing numbers from his information sheet into the appointment computer. He's looking at his watch and, desperately, at me.

I sigh. I look up at the secretary, still typing in numbers.

"Go ahead," I say finally. "I'll call and give you the appointment."

He smiles gratefully and bolts.

I make the appointment for Friday afternoon, call and let him know, then spend the intervening days agonizing over how this is going to work, whether there's a way to pull it all together for him, have it all make sense to him. Making sure he comes in, he gets the tests, he co-operates with what needs to be done—that is a fundamental part of my job.

On Friday afternoon, lifting his chart from my pile, I feel a sudden rush of anxiety. I explain the situation to my attending: about Pulmonary clinic, about the TB test and the X-ray and the smoking and the "irrelevant" problem of the fumes.

"Look," I say. "I'm frustrated. I feel like he's got one agenda, and the pulmonary people have another, and communication just isn't happening."

"What's your agenda?" my attending asks.

A pause. I haven't really thought about this before. Doesn't it seem as if we have too many agendas here already? The last thing we need is for me to have one, too. . . . I laugh at my subconscious thought processes.

"I think the smoking's really important," I say, slowly. "To him, and to his lungs—whatever else is happening with them."

The attending nods.

"I think we have to address the question of the fumes, even if it's not part of his pulmonary problem, because it's a big issue to him and by ignoring it we lose credibility."

He nods again.

"But I don't know how to do that," I add.

He thinks for a minute. "You could send him to Occupational Medicine, and they can investigate it. That's their job."

I feel like a huge weight has just been lifted off my shoulders. "Really?" Of *course*. Perfect.

"Okay," I say. "And the third thing is his pulmonary fibrosis, which needs to be worked up, but in a way that's intelligible to him. Those three things are my agenda."

"Great," he says. "Go with it."

"One other thing—" I say.

"Yes?"

"So Pulmonary wants to do all this fancy stuff—a spiral CT, for instance. And I don't get it. The results will be interesting, but what will it really accomplish? It seems like all the things we're looking for we'd treat about the same. Will it change our management?"

He sighs. "I don't know," he says. "But I'm not a pulmonologist. You can ask them that. But they're good guys; they know what they're doing. If they want it, it probably makes sense."

I nod.

"You don't have to understand everything that happens in their heads. You just have to guide him through it."

Okay, I think. I can handle that.

DURING HIS VISIT, we spend a long time talking about smoking. The counseling techniques I learned in medical school come back to me gradually as we work through the process. We set a quit date, talk about which cigarettes are hardest for him to give up, ways to distract himself. We discuss what to expect, what was hardest for him last time. I ask about support structures: "Does your wife smoke?" I ask.

"No," he says.

"Will she be supportive of your stopping?"

He sighs, looks away from me. Then looks back, grimacing. "I hate to say this—but she's really not supportive of anything. It's been awful, for years. . . . I think that's a lot of what's wrong with my life."

I nod slowly.

"Have you thought about ways of dealing with that?"

"I suppose someday I'll have to get out of it—but I don't think I'm able to right now."

I nod again. "That's very hard," I say sincerely. And then, when he doesn't seem inclined to elaborate, I steer the conversation quietly to other topics. This is one of the things I am trying to learn; there are times when it's enough just to listen. I don't have to come up with solutions to all his problems—I can't. But I also don't have to.

I put a lot of time into trying to explain to him why the pulmonary tests are so important. The visceral resistance is powerful—he knows what's wrong with his lungs, it's the fumes, and the smoking, and our silly CTs aren't going to help anything. But if I'll work with him on his agenda, he seems willing to accept my emphasis on mine.

I PRESENT TO my attending, who agrees enthusiastically with the plan, and comes back in with me for the final bit of the conversation. We go over details that need to be ironed out; one of them is the mechanics of getting a nicotine patch, which the patient has decided would be helpful.

"If you pay for it," I explain, "you can get it right away; but it will be expensive. Or, I can order it for you, which will make it free, but you'll have to wait for four to six weeks."

He nods.

"We can do it either way," I say. "Which do you think would be better?"

He opens his mouth to speak, then makes a gesture of frustration. "You—" He stops, then starts again. "You are my doctor. I have told you everything; I will not hold anything back from you. I will do whatever you say is best—but you must decide. I put myself in your hands."

He ends this little speech and looks at me expectantly.

I feel a part of myself recoil in fear and panic and denial—no. I can't be your doctor. You don't understand, I'm only an intern—worse yet, I'm a fraud. I don't know anything. . . . Get out, run, go find yourself a real doctor!

And I feel the impulse to turn to my attending, that kindly, authoritative presence, so familiar in form if not in specifics; to give him the brief, uncertain glance which would signal him to take over the interview, unobtrusively, knowing that it wasn't going the way I wanted it to—

Instead I hear my voice, clear and steady. "I prefer to look at it differently," my voice is saying. "This is a partnership. You and I will work together to find what is best for you, and do it. I will give you my information and opinions. You will give me your perspectives on what will work best for you. We will make a plan together. Ultimately, it is your life. Especially with something like stopping smoking, you will have to do most of the work. But I will be here to help you and support you in every way I can. We'll work on it together—"

He thinks for a minute; and then he smiles broadly, nodding enthusiastically. "Yes," he says. "A partnership. That's good."

My attending stands up and steps toward the door. "Excuse me, I'm going to go now."

The patient turns to him. "You're leaving me?" he asks jokingly.

"I leave you in good hands," he says, and flashes a warm, approving smile at me as he steps out the door.

I smile in return to thank him, not the thanks of a student to a teacher but of a junior to a senior colleague, one doctor to another.

We close the visit, agreeing that he'll call me in a week, a few days after he plans to quit smoking, to give me an update. We'll meet again a week or so later.

"Any questions?" I ask.

He shakes his head.

"I'm taking my CNA exam in a couple of weeks," he offers suddenly. "Someday I would like to be a nurse."

"Wow," I say. "That's great."

"I want to help people," he says earnestly.

"Good luck," I say.

"Thank you," he says.

4. Night Float

Sleeping with a pager is an exercise in suspended disbelief, a triumph, as the joke goes about second marriages, of optimism over experience. Persuading your system that it is worthwhile, or even possible, to sleep in spite of the probability, almost certainty, of being unpleasantly roused in a short time, is no simple task.

Lying on the cot of my call room, I curl around the little black box, its plastic body barely touching my stomach. Even though it is a primary instrument of torture for me as an intern, I have a certain paradoxical affection for my pager. I keep it on the beep/vibrate setting; it chirps for a while and then vibrates. It seems to me a wriggly, excitable beast; almost puppyish.

I've spent a lot of time lately thinking about pagers, and about sleep. I'm doing "night float," working 8:00 P.M. to 8:00 A.M. doing "cross-cover"—looking after patients for the interns who have gone home—and doing the night admissions. In the morning I hand over the admitted patients to the regular teams, who will take over responsibility for their care. This system was created to improve working conditions for medical residents, to ease the long shifts and sleepless nights. We have it in only one of the four hospitals I'll work at in this program, the private hospital. At the others, the university and VA and county hospitals, we do traditional overnight call every fourth night, thirty-six hours of continuous work without help. At this hospital, the night float team lets the regular teams rest.

"Float" is a curiously appropriate term. I feel as if I were floating, in many ways. Part of it comes from the surreal quality of the hospital at night, accentuated by the fact that for these weeks I seldom see daylight, and when I do it is the blinding glare of midmorning when I am sleepiest. Overall, though, the floating sensation has less to do with nights than with my role. I don't have patients who are mine. I admit them and hand them off, baby-sit the cross-cover folks and return them to their primary teams. I don't have a sense of belonging, of investment, of responsibility; I'm not grounded, I'm floating. It's a strange feeling.

On this particular night, I manage to settle down for a nap at around 4:00 A.M. My pager explodes at four-thirty.

"Admission, for you," says my resident's voice on the other end of the line as I sleepily answer the page. "Large hemorrhagic CVA. Eighty-two-year-old. I'll meet you in a couple minutes on the floor."

THE PATIENT IS lying in his bed, unable to speak, making occasional strangled sounds. The right side of his body is arched back, limbs rigid, toes pointed. This is called decerebrate posture, an indication of severe damage deep in the brain. A bad sign.

I get the history from his wife, who is advanced in age but looks healthy, though terribly afraid. They celebrated their fiftieth wedding anniversary the year before.

"About two in the morning, we were talking and suddenly he just keeled over—"

We go through the story, then something suddenly strikes me: "You were up, talking?"

"Yes."

Reality check. "Are you often up at two in the morning?" I ask, curious.

"Yes," she says.

I nod. "Okay."

"We stay up late, we sleep late," she adds, hanging her head.

"That's fine," I say, smiling. "I was just checking."

More questions, piecing together his previous history (he's been incredibly healthy, until tonight), his social history, his health habits.

"Does he smoke?"

"No. We both quit ten years ago."

I nod.

"Alcohol?"

"Just a glass of wine sometimes. We'll play some cards, have a little wine. In fact, we were going to have a glass of wine this evening. . . ." She looks stricken.

There's a pause. "This must be terribly hard for you," I offer gently after a moment.

"Just give me my husband back," she says. "I don't care if he's crippled, paralyzed, whatever; just so long as he has some part of his mind. I want him back." She stares at him, sleeping now in the bed. "Fifty-seven years," she says.

I'm not sure what to say or do; what does one answer, to emotions like these? I don't know what's going to happen. I can't reassure her that he will be all right, even that he won't die. On the other hand, I can't help her start to grieve, because it isn't clear yet what she would be grieving over. Her whole life will almost certainly be radically changed starting tonight, but I don't know how, so I can't help her to prepare.

I rub my sleepy eyes. She seems to have forgotten that I'm there. She simply watches him.

I TALK WITH his attending, who is obsessed by the idea that there is some obscure secondary cause for his stroke, that he has amyloidosis maybe, that we should be doing a biopsy of his rectum. I'm dubious and he sounds offended; "I'm just trying to make things interesting," he says.

I write the admission note and orders that will set things in motion until the team takes over in the morning.

A COUPLE OF hours later, I find myself in the hospital cafeteria, grabbing a cup of coffee before morning signout. One of the other interns, a day person, is sitting at a table, and waves at me as I walk in.

"Hey." I smile at him wearily.

"Was it a busy night?"

"Not too bad. Lots of cross-cover. Just one admission."

"What's the admit? I'm on today, I'll probably get it."

"Just a stroke," I say.

He cocks an eyebrow, as well he should: "Just?"

"I'm sorry," I say. "I don't mean it like that. Not 'just' for him, but 'just' for us—not a lot to do: watch him mostly, hope he gets better."

I GO HOME and sleep for most of the day. In the early evening, before I have to be at work, I go to the gym with another intern, Chris. We have a deal with each other. We force each other to go work out at least once every few days, as call schedules allow. We pit our energies for a change against simple combatants, struggling with iron instead of blood. Between measured heavy breaths we talk about work (names omitted, of course), vent sorrows, frustrations, anger. Chris is working in the Intensive Care Unit, he has patients whom he's never seen move, much less speak.

"I have this fifteen-year-old-kid," he says, "a near drowning. His little sister was actually drowning, and he swam in to get her. She's fine, and he's going to die. The family won't speak to her. They say, 'We *told* you not to swim there.'"

There's a pause while he concentrates on bench-pressing, face red, breaking a sweat.

"The sister's only eleven," he adds. "How long do you think before we'll be admitting her on psych or neuro with an overdose?"

There's nothing I can say.

After lifting, I shower, exchange my sweats for scrubs, add a white coat, and head to work. The intern with whom I had breakfast is sitting at the desk in the unit, and looks up as I come in.

"That guy you admitted with the stroke?"

"Yeah?"

"He died."

Time stops for a second.

"Oh," I say.

"This afternoon," he says.

"Was it—" I hesitate. "Was there anything I should have done differently?" I ask, carefully.

"I don't think so," he says.

Funny that that should be my first response—not, Oh God, I'm sorry, but, Was it my fault?

I think for a minute.

"His wife?" I ask. "She must be devastated."

"I think she's okay," he says. "I mean—she was very upset, obviously. But I think she was happy with how things went, at the end."

I nod. "Good."

I feel numb. I feel a hard, clear wall in my head shielding me against emotional involvement. Where did this come from? Am I just too tired? Or has it changed me, being an intern?

I'm not really sad for him, not much. He had just what I, what many people, would hope for: to be perfectly healthy to a ripe old age, and then drop dead all of a sudden, no prolonged illness or suffering, just one day there and the next gone.

But his wife—I should be able to hurt for his wife. I feel a thick, hard ache in my chest, but I'm not sure if it's for her or for me.

LATER THAT NIGHT, around 3:00 A.M., I'm in bed, catching a half hour of precious sleep, when my pager goes off. I go through the usual routine of swatting at it until the beeping stops, turn on the bedside lamp, dial the number.

"This is the intern on cross-cover, answering a page."

"Hi. This is Susan, on Four West. I'm just calling to notify you that your patient died."

I absorb the words in disbelief. This is a joke, right? A joke or a nightmare. It doesn't really happen like this, someone casually paging to say, Your patient died. This can't be real.

"It's Mr. Pirelli," she says.

I have the overhead light on now, and my glasses propped skewed half falling from my nose and I'm grabbing for my signout sheet—but suddenly I recognize the name, and things fall into place. He was a comfort-care-only patient, the decision had been made to withdraw care except to keep him comfortable. They were waiting for him to die, and now he has. That's why I didn't get an earlier call. There was nothing more to do.

I'm still holding the phone. My adrenaline-revved heart is pounding.

"I'm sorry," I say finally, breaking the pause. "I've never done this before. Can you tell me what I'm supposed to do?"

The nurse laughs in a friendly way. "Usually, you call the attending. And you can write the note saying there are no respirations, and so on; or we can. Either way."

"I'll come up there," I say.

I GO TO see him, out of some strange sense of balance perhaps, because I wasn't there to see my own patient die.

The family is gathered in the room. Six or eight of them are there, his children and grown grandchildren, standing close together in a supportive circle of grief and comfort. They step aside as I enter, to let me do my momentary task. "I'm sorry," I say.

"It's okay," they answer, and some manage to smile gently. They all look as if they'll be all right. The death was expected; they were prepared; and they have each other. I am relieved. They don't need me.

I step to the bedside. There he is, mouth open, still and silent. I remember being up much of the night with him a week or so ago, fussing over his respirator settings, the crackles and wheezes in his lungs that wouldn't clear. He looks just the same yet totally different; a puppet without a hand, a waxwork, an empty shell. I bend to listen to his chest, to feel for the absent pulse. His body is still warm.

I write the death note, call the attending ("I'm just calling to notify you"), fill out some paperwork. Then go back to my call room to lie down, waiting for the pager to go off again.

Through the rest of the night and the day that follows, I find myself avoiding eating anything with my fingers, as if my hands had death on them, and I couldn't wash it off. I touched a dead man this morning. He was still warm.

5. Crying

The ups and downs of internship are rapid and severe. One minute I feel like a "real" doctor, albeit a young and inexperienced one, the next minute I feel like a complete idiot. Sometimes I can't imagine how I got this far, I don't think I'll be able to get through the day or hour, much less a year of internship and a life as a doctor.

The moments that are bad for me are strangely timed. I detect a pattern to them, but not the one I would have expected. Overload and not emotional upset tends to get to me. I'm fine with crises or blowups, less so with the mounting masses of low-intensity detail work. I find expectation, rather than reality, hardest to manage. I'm always more tired going into a thirty-six-hour shift, the "on-call" day, than coming out of it, "postcall," or just "post." I'm more stressed when I'm waiting for an admission than when I'm working on one.

By these criteria, it is not surprising that I should sense a certain fragility in my psyche from the beginning of my last shift on night float. I switch from there to day work in the same hospital, on the general medical service or "ward service." My last night on float will meld into my first morning on the day team. I'm picking up a huge collection of very sick people from an intern who is leaving. I've seen a lot of this intern while I've been on float. She's almost never gone by 8:00 P.M. when I arrive, and she always looks stressed and tired. I'm not looking forward to taking over her job.

I'm hoping that things will be quiet tonight, that I'll have time to have a look at my new patients' charts, read through their notes, get a sense of what's going on before I take over the service. And I could use a little sleep. The idea of taking over this large and complicated team exhausted from the start is terrifying.

For the first few hours of the night, I'm busy with cross-cover. At midnight, when things are starting to settle, I retreat to my call room to make up data sheets on my new patients. I try to reassure myself, it will be okay . . .

Then my pager goes off. The display shows my resident's number; "Admission for you, coming in from the ER—AIDS patient with two days of severe headache and intractable vomiting."

I swing into motion, collect my coat, my stethoscope, and head to the floor. I don't run, but I always seem to walk fast, hurrying, in the hospital; I feel chronically rushed, a consequence of never being entirely in control.

I see the patient, gather his history, examine him. He lies uncomfortably in the bed. His neck is stiff and his eyes extremely photophobic; he's wearing sunglasses in the middle of the night amid the dim lights of the ward. When I have to check the reflexes of his pupils, he recoils from my penlight. He's coherent but exhausted, keeps dropping off to sleep midsentence. He looks very ill.

His partner hovers close by, wildly anxious, providing tangential information in voluminous detail, needing constant support and reassurance.

As I'm leaving the room, my pager goes off. "There's another one for you," my resident says. "End-stage liver disease. I'll get started on it, you finish up there, okay?"

"Okay," I answer.

As I'm gathering my thoughts, there's a tap on my shoulder. The patient's attending has come in to see him despite the late hour. She's a family practice doctor. She explains that she doesn't have many AIDS patients, and she's very unsure of what to do. Her suggestions to me are peppered with pauses and uncertainties: "Well—we could—" "And I guess we have to think about . . ." "But I don't know."

"They did a CT without contrast from the ER, but we might want to repeat it, with contrast this time. . . . Or maybe we don't have to? But probably we should, I guess. You could do it tonight—or in the morning. I guess either one is okay. . . . Whatever you guys think—"

Sometimes attendings will say, "You decide," or, "Do what you think is best," in a way that connotes that they've thought it out, that either one is acceptable, and that they should build your clinical skills by making you decide. This attending clearly isn't sure what to do, and this fact fills me with an unfamiliar depth of panic.

Just as we are finishing a long and slow discussion, my resident arrives, and it starts all over again. I watch the minutes tick away on the wall clock; minutes of potential sleep, minutes I needed to learn about my new team. "Well, I guess that would be all right," the attending is saying.

My resident, by contrast, knows exactly what she wants to do. Viral cultures, bacterial cultures, fungal cultures; gram stain of the CSF, VDRL, cryptococcal antigen, pneumococcal and meningococcal and h. flu antigen. Start antibiotics and antivirals, review the CT, order another CT, with contrast—morning is okay, the things we're looking for won't change too much before then.

She goes on: "They didn't check his opening pressure on the spinal tap—which means you'd better do a careful fundoscopic exam. Preferably with his pupils dilated; you can order atropine drops from the pharmacy to the floor."

I think of his cries of pain at the brief, not very bright flashes of light I used to test his pupils, imagine submitting him to a lengthy fundoscopic exam with his pupils dilated. Looking for papilledema, swelling of the optic disc. I've never seen papilledema. I know what it's supposed to look like but have no idea how hard it is to see. I don't know if I'd recognize it if it hit me on the head with a baseball bat. But I'm supposed to put him through this anyway.

My resident is still talking, adding to the list of things to do. I'm scribbling everything down as fast as I can on the sheet of paper in front of me, now completely filled with scratched notes and boxes. A hundred things to do, orders, calls to the lab, the pharmacy, the attending—

"His electrolytes are pretty abnormal, so we'll have to replete him. Give him potassium but not too much, because we don't know how his kidneys are doing. Calculate how much you want him to get and infuse it, but remember, you can't give over ten an hour IV, so figure out what volume you want him to get and how much to add, work out the different solutions and the rate—more at first probably with less K, to get his volume up, and then change over—"

I spend a few intense minutes calculating electrolyte volumes and concentrations and finally arrive at a set of solutions that will work.

My resident looks up. "I'm still worried about something fungal. Oh hell, you know, we'd better just go ahead and add amphoterocin. If it turns out he doesn't need it, we can just stop it in the morning."

My heart sinks. I'm not sure I can handle one more thing, but I nod, "Okay."

"But," she goes on, "keep a really close eye on his kidney function, 'cause we're giving him a whole bunch of nephrotoxins, and he could just crash. And of course we're giving him that CT with contrast—another nephrotoxin—in the morning. But we'll try, just watch him really, really closely."

What does this mean? I wonder. Am I supposed to be checking his renal function every two hours, every hour? But even those tests take a while to become elevated after the damage is done, so how am I supposed to do this? But she's racing on—

"He needs to be well hydrated with the ampho of course, give a five-hundred-cc bolus of normal saline before and again after the dose. And you know that ampho gets given over four hours. I'm not sure what volume of which solution it comes in though, so you'd better call and find that out, too—"

I stare at my careful calculations of exactly how much fluid we want him to get in how much time, how much potassium, and so on, and realize it's all just been invalidated by this extra element to the equation.

"And make sure to give a one-milligram test dose of the ampho first, to see if he'll tolerate it; then recheck his blood pressure and clinical status, and if he's all right, you can order to go ahead and give the rest—"

She's talking very fast, as if just reminding me of things I should already know; only I've never done any of this before. The only time I ever gave ampho was when I did infectious disease consults as a student, when we would write, "Suggest ampho" in the note, and that was all. I've never had to deal with the details.

It's the test dose of the amphoterocin that carries me over the edge. I feel the tears inexorably rising to my eyes. They're slow enough at first for my ducts to drain, I feel my eyes moisten, but they do not overflow. I hope that my resident and I will be able to pass off my sudden sniffling as an acute attack of allergies, or a developing cold. *I will not cry!* I will not cry at least until my resident is gone, or until I can make a saving dodge to the bathroom. But she's midsentence, and I can't do that now.

"Don't forget to call CT first thing in the morning to make sure that contrast scan gets done the minute they get here. You can lay a guilt trip on them; remind them that you didn't call them in in the middle of the night—"

In the back of my mind the thought: But first thing in the morning I'm going to be trying to figure out who the hell these other people are I'm supposed to be taking care of—

A renegade tear slips out my eye and spatters—I'm looking down at my to-do sheet—onto my glasses. My resident glances up at me, suddenly uncertain.

"Go on," I say.

She pauses a moment, then does as told. "And call Infectious Disease to get them involved. Henry Richmond, he's great, make sure to get him—"

I nod. More tears are chasing the first one now, but I am still able to hold the stream flowing down my cheeks separate from the rest of me, my voice is steady. "Anything else?"

She pauses. I see the sympathy, and the uncertainty, in her eyes. I'm new at being an intern, but she's equally new at being a resident. *I've never had an intern before, and suddenly I've got one and she's crying.* I don't think anyone taught her how to handle this.

"What can I do to help you?" she asks at last, gently.

Kindness is the final straw, breaking down my last defense as curtness perhaps would not have, and I begin to cry in earnest now, sobbing uncontrollably into cupped hands.

She rubs my shoulder gently for several minutes, until at last I regain enough control to be able to speak.

"I'm sorry," I sputter out helplessly.

She just shakes her head.

"I don't know what's happening—I don't usually do this. I'm okay, I just got—overwhelmed."

I try to explain: "I was already nervous from knowing I would be tired and picking up this big team, and I haven't done inpatient stuff in so long, and I was just a little—panicky. And somehow this—and the other person coming in at the same time—suddenly it was all just too much, and I just went into overload—" I stop, choking, to catch my breath after the rush of words. "I'm sorry. I'll be all right, really."

I frown, willing myself to be fine, though my eyes are betraying me. The tears start to roll again every time I open my mouth to speak.

"It sucks," she says quietly. "Internship—just sucks. And it can be completely overwhelming, and no one gives you a chance to feel that way."

She goes off to deal with the second admission, after sternly admonishing me to get this guy tucked in and then go have a snack, take care of myself for a bit. I do that—having food in my system is a remarkable boost—come back, recheck the orders, make the necessary calls, write up his note.

The next morning, having gotten a grand total of a half hour of sleep, I pick up my new team. The funny thing is, I do okay. I quickly get up to speed on the patients. I find that I know what I'm supposed to do, and I slog through the day's heavy workload, feeling busy and a little stressed but definitely in control. I watch myself, as if from above. I look confident, smart, and resilient. Solid. A good intern.

I wonder where she went, the self who was weeping uncontrollably at the nurses' desk a brief half day earlier. I wonder which of these is me at heart, or how it is possible to be both in such short succession. I feel the strength, the confidence, yet also the panic, lying somewhere close, not deeply hidden. I try to accept that this is how it will be, this segment of my life: awful and great and weak and strong. I work at savoring the good moment, knowing that tears are lurking out there, that the panic will surely be back before too long.

I will never learn as much in any year of my life as I will in this one. I may never have the same intensity of experience. I intend to make the most of it. At the same time, I cling to the knowledge that someday it will be over, that internship has to end. . . .

6. The Last Presentation

As we're lifting at the gym, I tell Chris, my fellow intern and exercise partner, the story of how I cried my last night on float.

"I cried on rounds once," Chris says suddenly.

His voice is strained. I look up. Usually we share our bad moments with each other, but he didn't tell me this story when it happened. I wonder if it was just too much to talk about.

"It was on the Intensive Care Unit. I had this woman who was dying. She was in DIC"—disseminated intravascular coagulation, an often fatal disorder where the blood first clots too much and then becomes unable to clot, leaving patients with terrible bleeding—"she was bleeding out of everywhere. She had blood coming out from her urinary catheter, her nasogastric tube, her endotracheal tube; she was oozing and bleeding out her IV sites, her central line, her A-line. It was awful. She'd been going down this path for days, it was just getting worse and worse—"

I nod gently. The pain is thick in his eyes and voice.

"It was time," he says. "Well—it was past time. But it was definitely time."

He pauses, then goes on.

"So we're on rounds. You know, unit rounds—"

I nod. Rounds in the Intensive Care Unit take forever. Instead of the usual quick presentation by the intern bringing the team up to date on the patient's condition and the previous day's events, ICU presentations are much longer and more formal. You begin with a summary of the last twenty-four hours' events, then a discussion of how the patient is feeling if he is well enough to tell you—which most aren't. Then you go through the full physical exam, ventilator settings, a dozen vital signs given in ranges across the day, thirty or more lab values, X-ray results, often EKG or other study findings. Then a full medication list, often twenty or thirty medications long. All this is just a prelude to the grand finale, the assessment and plan by system—respiratory, cardio-vascular, infectious disease, renal, endocrine, and so on, almost a dozen in all, a list of issues in each category, active or inactive, differential diagnoses, treatment plans.

"So the nurses keep grabbing me, saying, can you come, we need to have this thing over. It's killing the family, it needs to end—"

I nod. He frowns, his forehead tight.

"So finally I interrupt, and I say, can we go out of order here, and jump ahead to this patient? 'Cause this is important, we have to get this over with.

"And they look at me. . . . But finally, okay, we go ahead to the patient."

He pauses again.

"So we go in there, and we're all standing in a circle the way you do on rounds. And I say, 'The family wants to withdraw support.' But they're all standing there, in that circle, you know, looking at me. So finally I say, 'You want me to *present?*'

"And they nod. I mean—everybody knows all about this patient. We've been doing this for weeks. But okay. So I say, this is a seventy-year-old woman with blah blah blah. And on physical exam she's bleeding out of this this this this and this and she looks like shit and she's miserable, and on labs and everything else she's completely fucked up.

"And there she is, lying in the bed, blood all over the place. And the family's out in the hall crying. And every minute of this is just hell, pure hell, for everybody—for her, for them. But the team is all still standing there. Waiting. With that *look*. And finally I say: *'You want me to go through this by system?'*"

His voice cracks, squeaks up a pained, jarring octave as he repeats the words.

"And then I turned and walked out."

His brows are furrowed, his lips tight with intense concentration and suppressed emotion. He reaches for the lifting bar as if to bend the steel.

7. Near-Death Experience

Jimmy Dorn was a seventy-year-old man who had been in excellent health and stayed far away from both hospitals and doctors in his seven decades. He had never had chest pain in his life. Had he been in a position to think at all, one can only assume that he would have been quite surprised when his heart suddenly stopped, as he was pushing his stalled car into the garage one pleasant Sunday afternoon. Technically, his heart went into ventricular fibrillation. The net effect was that it stopped pumping blood.

Luckily for him, someone saw him fall; even luckier, that person happened to know CPR. After a few minutes of chest compressions and mouth-to-mouth breathing, an ambulance arrived and a triad of electrical shocks was enough to get his heart back into a normal rhythm. He arrived at the hospital awake, alert, and temporarily deprived of all short-term memory.

"Do you know why you're here?" I ask, knowing this was explained to him an hour or so earlier.

His face goes blank. "No," he admits.

"You've just had a cardiac arrest," I say. "Your heart stopped. Someone came and got it going again; but now we have to find out why it stopped, and do something about it, so it won't happen again. Do you understand?"

"Yes," he says.

"What year is it?" I ask him in the course of our interview.

"Well, how 'bout you tell me what year it is?" He has a warm southern accent.

"I'd like to have you try to tell me, first."

"Well, that's a tough one." He squints at me.

"Just guess," I suggest.

He thinks for a while. "1980?" he offers finally.

"That's pretty good," I say. "Would you believe me if I told you it was 1996?"

"No," he says. "Probably not."

I smile. I guess I won't, then. "Who's the president?" I ask.

"Clinton."

"Great," I say.

"I've asked all my questions," I say, at the end of the interview. "Now, do you have any for me?"

He thinks for a minute. "No."

"Okay," I say. "I'll see you a little later."

I've almost made it out the door when his voice stops me:

"Wait, I do have one question."

I turn back.

"What's that?" Carefully attentive.

"How old are you?" he drawls.

I laugh. "Twenty-five," I confess.

"Damn, they're making doctors young these days!"

I laugh again and leave.

I'M SIGNING OUT to the cross-cover intern when the overhead loudspeaker goes off. "Code Orange, room two seventy-nine—" This hospital has an unusual collection of alarm codes, including a "Code Seven" for a stolen baby. ("Go to the nearest window and look for a person carrying a baby. If you sight such a person, call security with your location immediately.") A Code Orange refers to an out-of-control patient. Room 279 is familiar, I realize with a sinking heart—that's Mr. Dorn's room.

My pager goes off at the same moment, and I dial the CCU, my fingers heavy. "So, what happened?"

"Mr. Dorn decided he wanted to leave."

Of course, I think to myself. He feels fine, and he can't remember minute to minute that he just had a cardiac arrest; so why would he want to stay?

"I'll be down there in a minute."

He's calmed down by the time I get there, sitting in the bed looking a little sheepish, having been told again about the situation. I talk with his family, and we arrange for one of them to be there at all times. I believe that this will solve the problem of his wanting to leave. They can keep explaining what's happened to him, and besides, he trusts them. If they say he ought to stay, he will.

I MAKE IT out of the hospital that night. The solution worked well, we had no further problems of his wanting to leave. I go to see him when I return in the morning, and we have another pleasant conversation.

"Where are you from?" I ask. There aren't many people with southern accents in Seattle.

"South Carolina. We came for a visit, and we just stayed. That was twenty-eight years ago."

"Wow," I say.

"Where did you do your training?" he asks me in turn.

"At Dartmouth, in New Hampshire."

"My daughter went to Dartmouth. Beautiful out there, in the fall," he says.

"Yes," I agree wistfully.

"Do you know why you're here?" I ask, after questioning him about symptoms, of which he still has none.

"My wife says my heart stopped, or something. I don't remember anything about it."

"Yes," I say. "That's right."

He nods wonderingly.

So he's imprinting memories, at least a little, now. I try to think of ways to test how well his memory is working.

"What did you have for breakfast?"

"Nothing worth eating." He grins charmingly. I smile back, recognizing that that didn't give me much information.

"Do you remember anything that happened yesterday?"

He thinks. "I was here, I think. . . ."

"Do you remember me?"

"A little." Is this a real "a little" or a polite "no," I wonder?

"How old am I?" I ask suddenly.

He looks startled by the question. "Pretty young, I'd say," he answers.

"Just checking," I say, unsure how to explain the question. His wife, who was there for the question the day before, smiles knowingly.

During the next few days, his memory improves. He still doesn't remember the actual arrest—he never will—but he knows that we told him it happened. His memory for new events goes back to normal. He knows me and the rest of the staff.

Meanwhile, he gets a coronary angiogram, which shows he has severe constriction in three major heart vessels. He'll have to have a bypass. His son-in-law, a doctor in town, wants a particular surgeon who works elsewhere and is away this week. Mr. Dorn will stay a couple days, then go to have the surgery done at another hospital.

We're mostly just watching him now, making sure he's stable until he gets the surgery. But I go in to chat with him once or twice a day.

"Your flowers are beautiful." He has a stunning arrangement of spring flowers.

"Aren't they nice? My son-in-law sent them. Did you notice the tulips? Hard to find this time of year. And the hyacinths. Spring flowers, in the fall."

"Which are your favorites?"

"Oh," he says, "I like all these, but my favorites are the roses." He plucks a fading flower neatly from the bouquet, then looks up. "I have over eighty kinds of roses in my garden."

"Really?"

He nods. "My son-in-law keeps bringing me more. He'd like to grow them himself, but he doesn't have the knack for it. His always die, so now he just finds ones he wants and brings them to me. I say, enough already! But secretly I love it." He smiles. I suspect his son-in-law has figured out the secret.

"My son-in-law is a doctor," he says, changing the subject. "Like you. Well—a nephrologist. I can't imagine being as dedicated to your work as you've got to be to be a doctor. He works twelve hours or more every day, goes in 'most every Saturday and Sunday, too. . . ."

"Mm," I say absently. "It can be a hard life."

"It ruined his first marriage," he says earnestly. "He has a daughter who's twenty-seven who hasn't spoken to him since the day she left for college. She just walked out the door and that was it. He was so busy being a doctor all the time he had nothing left to be a father too. But that's the kind of thing you have to do in a field like that—"

"I'm going to leave before you get me so depressed I quit," I say, grinning at him.

ON THE LAST morning before he's transferred, the assembled team goes to see him on rounds. We step in and look around the room for a moment, blinking in the bright sunlight streaming in the window, without seeing him. The bed and chair are empty. The bathroom door is open, but he's not in there.

As my eyes adjust I see him, finally. He's sitting up in the windowsill, knees tucked under his chin, looking pensively out over the concrete courtyard below. I've never seen a patient sit on the windowsill before.

We gather around him and he smiles benevolently at us. "Good morning."

"Good morning."

I take the lead: "How are you doing this morning?"

"Okay."

"Enjoying the sunshine?" It seems unfair not to acknowledge his choice of seating.

"Yes. It's a beautiful morning. The sunrise was just breathtaking."

Funny how easy it is to forget there's a world out there. Easy for me, feeling as if I live between these walls; how much easier for the patients, who really do. I look out at the blue sky dotted with fluffy clouds, the patches of green grass, the wildflowers, and feel a sudden lift, and a rush of gratitude to him for reminding me.

We have the requisite chat about his symptoms this morning and the day's game plan. "Anything else?" I ask, as we turn to leave.

"Well, there is one more thing—"

I see my resident glance at her watch. "What's that?" I know whatever he says will be interesting; I hope it won't be another quip about my age.

"Well, I keep thinking . . . The strangest thing is: the other day, you know? I *died*."

I nod. His voice is full of awe.

"I was dead for a couple of seconds, and then I came back."

I nod again, but something in his manner says he hasn't reached his point yet. He frowns.

"You know how people say they're supposed to see things—the light at the end of the tunnel, or their life flashing before their eyes, or something?"

"Yes . . ."

"Only I don't remember anything about it."

He looks simply crestfallen.

He stops, and I peer at him. "Mr. Dorn," I say after a moment, "Are you disappointed that you missed out on your near-death experience?"

He squints up at me. "Well, yes, I suppose I rather am."

He sighs, looks out the window. "Do you think the people who say that are making it up? Or did I just forget?" He shakes his head, sadly.

I watch him for a minute, framed in the bright light of the window, comfortably perched, surrounded by his beautiful flowers, the brows over his blue eyes furrowed in thought. I try to think of something to say and can't. So I just smile, and shake my head.

"I'm sure you'll figure it out."

"I s'pose."

He smiles at me.

"We've got to go," I say regretfully.

"I know you do." He shakes his head and sighs, then waves us off. As we file out, a procession of starched coats, I see him turn back to the window, his figure washed in a halo of white light.

8. Code 199

Walking down the hallway, immersed in thoughts of work, I hear the slight crackle of the PA system turning on. Amazing how you can learn to orient to a slight detail in a sea of stimuli if that one thing is important enough. Usually the PA's message is irrelevant to me, but every once in a while it's critical. My body tenses, on hold for the second between the crackle and the announcement.

"Code one ninety-nine," comes the voice. "Room six twenty-five E."

These are the words I'm always half listening for, the ones that mean *run.*

No word in medical language is so fraught with meaning as this unassuming one: *code.* We use it, of course, in the usual sense: "Do the orthopedists write in code?—I can't read a word of their notes." Then there are the emergency codes I mentioned earlier, the Code Oranges and Browns, fires and hazardous-material spills and unruly visitors. And there's another vast category of codes related to billing, which I hardly bother with as a resident but which will occupy huge amounts of my time later on.

All these pale beside our overriding usage of the term: a "code" means a death, and everything that surrounds it. More specifically, it means a cardiopulmonary arrest—a stoppage of the heart or breathing. There's a protocol for how to try to bring someone back from this, laid out in a training program called ACLS: advanced cardiac life support. You study it for the first time in medical school, and again as an intern. You learn the pathway by rote: A, B, C: airway, breathing, circulation. Check first: is the patient breathing? Does he have a pulse? If not, the code begins. CPR, oxygen, IV lines, a breathing tube into the throat, a cardiac monitor to show the electrical rhythm of the heart. Then electric shocks in escalating strengths, then a series of medications, then . . . and so on. The process can last anywhere from a few minutes to more than an hour. "A code" refers to all of this, from the moment of alert until you either get the patient back or declare him gone.

"To code" becomes a verb in two senses. In reference to a patient, "to code" means to die, to have a cardiac or pulmonary arrest. "It was almost the end of the surgery and suddenly he just coded." At first this phrasing seemed strange to me. It sounded as if people did it on purpose, the way we say "She failed chemotherapy" as though it were a character flaw. Soon the phrase became familiar and ceased to bother me.

"To code" applied to a doctor means to try to get someone back from death. I emphasize "try," because the numbers are against; 80 percent of in-hospital codes end unsuccessfully.

"Calling a code" also has two meanings, ironically different. The first person on the scene, the person who finds the patient pulseless or not breathing, "calls a code" to initiate the process. The announcement for a "Code 199" is made. The people assigned to handle such crises—usually the medicine team on call, plus specially trained nurses and a respiratory technician, perhaps a surgeon or anesthesiologist—come running. If the code is unsuccessful, the person in charge calls to end the code, to declare death. So a code is called twice: once at the beginning, once at the end.

As THE WORDS crackle over the intercom, my body is already in movement. I run, in this case, up six flights of stairs, fast, my legs protesting the sudden exercise. I fight the impulse to linger just slightly, not wanting to be the first one there. This is, in fact, what happens. I burst out of the stairwell door on the sixth floor, an unfamiliar place, the rehab ward, I later learn. Someone points me toward the room. There she is on the bed, no IV line, no resuscitation equipment. And no other doctors. No one. Whoever called the code must have run to get help or equipment. Just a still figure in a bed and me.

My worst nightmare as a physician is not about giving the wrong antibiotic, missing some allergy or drug interaction, and having someone die because of an order I carelessly wrote—though it could happen, and it does terrify me. It's not missing a diagnosis, something I should have known and was too tired to think of, something I didn't know but would have if I'd read more journals, paid more attention in medical school. Nothing so complex as that, but simply this: to be the first person on call to a code, there in a room with—with what? A body that's coding? A person who's dying? What do all these words and images mean? But, there with—my fingers above an artery, and to be unable to determine whether there is a pulse.

You would think this would be so easy. You would think that, in a world so full of vagaries, this one thing would be pristine: a heartbeat or no heartbeat.

The truth is a pulse is a tenuous thing. Is that a flutter of faint motion below your questing finger, is it a movement transmitted from one of the many others who may be pushing, compressing, ventilating—so many big and little jerks and movements, against which background to seek out that tiny life beat? Is it your imagination, creating a burst where there is none, seeking so hard it finds what isn't there? Is it your own artery pinched against the patient's skin so that you feel your pulse as hers? This happens, very readily. You could feel a pulse in a stone wall.

Or, alternatively, are you slightly in the wrong spot and so don't feel a real pulse, then declare a false catastrophe? Is it all, as you may wonder and will often wish, just a mistake, a foolish thing gone wrong, an overreaction? There are times when you listen to the chest of someone who is walking and talking and can't hear a heartbeat. You know it's there, but for some reason it eludes you. If that has happened before, how can you know it isn't happening now?

Since becoming a doctor, I have developed a nervous habit of holding my own radial pulses; mapping them out, the course of the artery, the spaces where it booms most brightly. I have a vague idea of doing an arterial blood draw on myself someday, drawn by some combination of machismo, simple curiosity, masochism, and a certain need to demonstrate the physical reality of my own anatomy—yes, I have an artery there, if you enter it you will hit blood.

These thoughts flicker half formed through my mind as I am deciding that no, I do not believe there is a pulse. I spin on the nurses who are appearing at the door, and say, We need a monitor, a face mask, IV access—

And then there is the rush of relief as, only seconds behind me, my senior resident appears, the blessed face of higher authority. I step back to roles with which I am comfortable, doing instead of thinking, following instead of leading. I step into position to start CPR, feeling suddenly calm. It occurs to me, unexpectedly, that I like CPR. I like to do compressions because it makes me feel useful. My arms are strong. I feel competent at that.

We start into the now-familiar rhythms of this process. I remember my first code, remember how it felt to watch someone die for the first time. I find myself comparing this to that day, remembering the shock and overload at being, for the first time, a witness to—a participant in—the death of a human being. Two years later a dead body, limp and motionless, is no longer a foreign thing; it is almost routine. A code feels less a person's death than a code: a strange, codified entity, a thing unto itself. I look at this body, and I can't do it, I cannot make myself feel what I felt that first time.

I study the body. Study "it," study "her"? My ongoing uncertainty of words seems to signify a deeper uncertainty of meaning. I have seen so many bodies, living and dead. I feel her chest under my compressing hands. I help to lift her so a shock pad can be stuck against her back. Touching her, I think, irrationally, of lovers whose skin I have delighted in, clasped beneath my fingers, massaged, caressed. What framework can I find to encompass both these concepts, the thrilling touch of beloved flesh, and this strange doughy substance beneath my hands?

What is skin, what are bodies?—these fragile, mortal shells that house us, all so much the same.

The minutes pass, half an hour, three-quarters; my resident carries us down the algorithms of ACLS. As each successive intervention proves unsuccessful, as her heart continues to refuse to beat, the chances of her surviving the code drop lower, finally down to nothing. Awareness settles, slowly. We continue for a while, against hope; finally my resident sighs. "Let's call it—"

We stop. There is the strange moment that follows, part sorrow, part relief. The body lies still now on the bed, becoming cold, tubes and needles emerging from it everywhere. What to do next?

I've gained a certain kind of power and insight in the years since my first code, and one of its strongest manifestations is the courage to follow where my instinct takes me. I no longer think: Is a person in my position supposed to do this? If it feels right to stay and clean her up, I'll do that.

So I stay, to pull the tube out of her throat, to throw away the syringes and the stickers and the pads. To cover her with a blanket, fold her hands across her chest, lift her head onto a pillow to make her look more comfortable. Preparing her for the daughter who is on her way, who will be here soon to say good-bye.

AND THEN—THIS is the perversity of medical life—I have to go to dinner. "Have to," because the cafeteria closes in five minutes. If I don't run down there now, I won't have any food all night, and I know that I need to eat to be physically strong enough to get through.

We sit, my resident and I, pushing salad around on our plates, trying to choke down bites of desperately needed nutrition but profoundly repelled by the idea of food. We make feeble attempts at conversation, then lapse into thoughtful silence. My pager goes off a few times, small detail calls. We've chosen a table by the wall telephone, so I can reach back to answer pages without disrupting the meal.

Then, mercifully, there is a little respite. My notes are done, our next admission is expected but hasn't yet arrived. My resident goes off to make a phone call and I wander, aimlessly, back to my call room. I sit down on the bed. A moment of free time is so unusual I don't know quite how to spend it—I shiver, cold.

Then, with sudden unexpected clarity, I know what to do. I strip out of my scrubs quickly, and step into the shower, setting my pager on the sink. I lean against the shower wall and feel the water flowing over me, warm and comforting, enveloping me. I scrub my skin and let the water carry away the sweat, the dirt, the lingering film of death that seemed to cover me.

I feel a sudden surge of pride and love for my body, my strong arms, long swimmer's legs, flat stomach. I admire my veins running resilient and blue-purple under my skin, my long, piano-playing fingers. I've often wondered what it is that carries me to the gym, on so many weary nights, the one consistent routine in my tired, chaotic, and desperately time-crunched schedule. Why do I choose exercise over sleep, food, sometimes friendship? I sense that because I am surrounded by disease and decay and death, I feel an urgent need to be strong, to be healthy. Youth and strength and overabundant health are my guarantors, my guards, the things that separate me from the tragedy all around me. My totem against the medical world's ugliness is insisting that my own body be beautiful.

I towel dry and dress, feeling human again, ready to face the night.

9. Mary Ann

There are certain little old women you simply can't help falling in love with. I knew this was one such the moment I saw her, sitting daintily on her ER gurney with her white sheet tucked neatly around her lap. She was tiny, old and frail, with angelic blue eyes and a sweet face. But there was something about her smile, something sparkly, almost mischievous, at moments. She calmly answered my questions about the stroke she'd apparently had the day before, which she'd just come in for this morning.

"I was sitting there and suddenly my whole left side wasn't working. My arm, my leg, nothing. Even my mouth felt strange. Not painful, just not working. I figured it was probably a stroke. I just sat there; I didn't know what to do—"

"You live alone?"

"Yes."

She sighs. "I could move my arm a little, that was all. I couldn't walk, even with Mary Ann to help me."

I frown slightly. I thought she lived alone? But Mary Ann must be her daughter. She probably said that, and I just wasn't listening properly.

"Are you able to walk on your own usually?"

"Oh, yes. Mary Ann and I, we get along pretty well."

Maybe she's a home health aide, not a daughter. I'm about to ask, but she goes on.

"I slept the whole night in the chair; I couldn't figure out how to get to the bed. So finally this morning, I gave my daughter a call and told her to come. She put me and Mary Ann in the car and drove us up here."

A different problem has caught my attention now. I try to formulate my next question carefully. "Did it occur to you at all to have someone bring you in last night, instead of waiting until this morning?"

"Well—my daughter's been in a bad mood, these past few days." She shakes her head. "I think maybe she's on her period." She glances up, as if to gauge the impact of this startling comment, then leans toward me and whispers conspiratorially: "I hate to say this, but she's a real bitch when she's on her period." She grins at me, giggles naughtily for a moment, then composes herself, folding her hands primly in her lap.

"So . . ." I've completely lost my train of thought. "So."

After my exam, I explain that we'll be admitting her to the neurology floor upstairs. We'll be doing some tests, keeping a close eye on her. Her daughters are welcome to visit.

"Can Mary Ann come up with me?" she asks promptly.

"I don't think there would be a problem with that," I say slowly, still not sure who this Mary Ann person is.

"Good," she says. She makes a gesture toward the corner of the room, which at first I don't understand. Then, in a sudden flash of comprehension, I realize that "Mary Ann" is her walker.

My God, I think. This woman is psychotic, and I didn't even realize it. This can happen. You're having what seems like a reasonable conversation with someone until some little thing strikes you as strange, and then you discover that she thinks it's 1962 and Nixon is president and two plus two is five.

I run through a bunch of questions, and she does fine. She really seems to make pretty good sense, apart from this funny fixation on her personified walker.

An ER nurse pops her head in the door. "They're ready to take her up whenever you're done."

"Okay," I say. "I'll just be a minute."

"Make sure Mary Ann comes up, too," my patient says. "I don't want her getting lost."

"Okay," I say, glancing at the nurse. "I'll make sure we bring her."

I'm on my way out the door, still puzzled, when suddenly I stop, turn back.

"Can I ask one more question?"

"Sure," she says.

"Why do you call your walker Mary Ann?"

She smiles, and rearranges her sheet on her lap before she answers. "Several years ago, my doctor and I realized that I was going to need to use a walker. We picked out this one, and my doctor said: 'It's going to be with you for the rest of your life, so you might as well name it.' So I did. Mary Ann has been a faithful companion to me, she has." She twinkles at me.

"I see," I say, smiling back. She's been trying to share the joke with me all along, wondering whether I would get it, and I almost didn't. Now she gives me a quick, approving nod, and I know I passed the test.

10. Deathwatch

You would think it would have been a conversation to remember. Charles Carson was a very young man, just turning forty, and he was dying. He'd been diagnosed a few months earlier with hepatocellular carcinoma (hepatoma, for short), related to his alcoholic cirrhosis and hepatitis C. It was the same disease my first clinic patient had, who had just died a few weeks earlier. It can't be treated and kills people quickly. We both knew he didn't have much time. He came in with a gastrointestinal bleed, his second big episode in a few weeks. He had esophageal varices, engorged veins in his throat from the blood backed up behind his liver, which bleed easily and terribly. His blood didn't clot well, because the liver couldn't do its work of making clotting enzymes.

I admitted him to the Intensive Care Unit, where we had the talk that I would try to recall somewhat later, but about which, for some reason, I am able to remember almost nothing beyond the impersonal details recorded in his admission note. We talked about the cancer, when and how it was diagnosed; about the bleeding, when it started, how much, all the gory details. And surely about other things. I know we discussed his alcoholism and recovery a little. I remember his telling me that he worried about his sponsees—I recall smiling at the word—in AA, about how they would manage when he was no longer there.

I remember he seemed nice. Maybe that was why I blocked out the rest; maybe I was too tired for another heartbreak.

He was seen by the gastroenterologists, who knew him well. We gave him octreotide, a drug that constricts the esophageal vessels, and the bleeding stopped, or at least slowed. "Try to get him home quickly," his primary doctor said. "He doesn't have much time left, and every day that he can spend at home instead of here is a blessing."

We transfer him out of the ICU, agree that if he's stable for another day he should go home. The first sign of trouble happens that afternoon.

A nurse comes up to me while I'm at the desk writing notes. "You know Mr. Carson?"

"Sure. Why?"

She frowns. "I'm not sure if he's crazy, or what—he's in there praying."

I go in and he is, indeed, murmuring fervent and feverish-sounding prayers. He stops when I come in. "Are you okay?"

He nods.

I'm not sure if this is normal or strange behavior. I don't know him well, and I also don't know how anyone should react, facing death at age forty. Maybe begging God for help makes sense. He seems lucid. I check his hands, which tremble slightly as he holds them forward; a sign of encephalopathy, brain injury. I start him on lactulose, the treatment for the brain toxicity induced by liver disease.

THE NEXT MORNING, I find him asleep and can barely wake him. I shake him vigorously and succeed in rousing him a little. "Ooh, baby—" he murmurs. I cannot get him to say anything else.

I read the note left by the cross-cover intern. He had become agitated then, gradually, less responsive during the course of the night. They increased the dose of his lactulose, then he became too confused to drink it. They tried to give it as an enema—the only other way to get it into the system, there is no intravenous equivalent—but he woke enough to fight them. A protracted struggle ended up in a huge mess, some bruised bodies and feelings, without the enema staying in long enough to be therapeutic.

A nurse appears at my shoulder and starts into a long explanation of why she doesn't want to try the enema again. He's scheduled for another dose this morning. "It's okay," I say with a heavy sigh. "It wasn't really helping anyway."

I go by his room a number of times that day. The "Ooh, baby—" that I heard this morning has become his mantra. He murmurs it softly in his sleep, or, when he occasionally becomes half-awake and agitated, screams it out over and over; "Ooh baby ooh baby OOH BABY . . ."

"Woo," he adds, occasionally, crowing. Some of the staff walking by titter, others wince. I am hurt, remembering him even in that brief initial encounter as a quiet, dignified man. He seemed like someone who would particularly not want to live out his last hours like this. Even if I was unable to do anything more substantive, I wish I could flip a switch in his brain that would cause him to say, "Holy Lord," or "Please" or "Help me!" instead.

It's after six that evening, I'm sitting at the desk finishing up a few notes when a nurse pulls on my arm. "The Carson family is here, and they want to talk to a doctor."

I glance at my watch. His attending came by a few hours ago and wouldn't be back. Both of my residents have gone home; I was hoping to be out soon myself. "Sure," I say. "I'll talk to them."

It's funny how quickly things change. Three months ago, I wouldn't have dreamed of holding a conference like this. Now it's difficult, but at the same time, a routine part of my job.

I meet the family—his brother, two sisters, and his girlfriend—and take them into the small room at the end of the hall where we hold meetings like this. It's small, but it has several comfortable chairs and lots of windows. I sit, and gesture for them to also.

I take a deep breath, and introduce myself. "Ideally I wouldn't be the one having this conversation with you. His attending doctors would, who have known him for a longer time, and who may know you a little, too. I'm sorry to be the one doing this, but I'm the only person here right now."

"Dr. White called, and explained the situation to us," the sister interjects, and I nod, relieved.

"'The situation,' meaning what?" the brother demands.

He looks accusingly at the sister, and then at me. Slowly, I begin. "As you know, Charles has a fatal cancer growing in his liver. There's nothing we can do to treat it or to save his life. He had a massive bleed into his gut a few days ago. He is absorbing certain toxins from that blood, nitrogen and other substances. Normally, his liver would be able to take the toxins out of his system. Since his liver is mostly destroyed by the cancer, it can't do that. The toxins are staying in his bloodstream and going to his brain, which is why he's acting this way."

I take a deep breath. "We have no way of treating that. The only drug we've got for it hasn't helped him. He probably isn't going to improve. We will do everything we can to make him comfortable, to make sure that he's not in any pain. But he probably has very little time left at this point."

My eyes shift from one to another of them as I talk, resting most often on his girlfriend. She's been here since this started, I know her best. Suddenly his brother breaks in, anger barely disguised in his voice: "Look," he says. "Why are you talking to her? You're supposed to be talking to all of us, but mostly you're looking at her. She's just his girlfriend. I'm his brother. I'm the blood relative. You talk to me."

"I'm sorry," I say, startled. "I was trying to talk to all of you equally. I'm very sorry."

"Look," he says. "No offense, but—"

I look up. No offense, but what?

"You're only an intern. I'd like to talk to one of his senior doctors."

"Of course," I say. Funny how, on the one hand, I think this is completely appropriate; on the other hand, that phrasing—"You're only an intern"—does actually offend me. Look, I want to say. Being *only* an intern means I spend twice the hours here that most senior doctors do, I know more about the patients than they do, and I put a hell of a lot more effort into their care. So by all means, talk to the attending; but don't "only" me. . . .

I swallow this sudden rush of thoughts, and police my tone carefully to filter out any hard edge. I wonder how much of my own inner hostility I am suddenly unleashing, how much more than the present situation I am tapping into.

"Of course," I repeat. "They're not here right now, but they'll be here in the morning. Or if you prefer, I can get you their numbers so that you can reach them before then."

"We have the number," his sister interjects. He looks up to frown at her.

"I want something from you," he says to me.

"Yes?" I say, warily.

"I want you to call them and get them to talk to me. I know it's hard to reach doctors. Since you are a doctor yourself, you'll have a better time than I will."

I frown. I have a lot to do. It's late, and I've been here for a lot of hours. Most of the work of getting in touch with attendings is waiting on the phone while their secretaries page them. He could spend that time as easily as I could. I'm not sure, among the many demands on my time, that this is an appropriate use of my energy.

"You say you have the number"—I nod toward the sister. "Have you tried just calling them?" If he's tried and not been able to get through, that's a different thing.

"I want you to call them for me," he repeats, not answering my question.

"I'm not sure that would make sense," I say, carefully.

"Are you willing to do it, or aren't you?"

"Look—" I begin.

"I don't want to dialogue about it. I just want to know: will you or won't you? If you refuse, fine."

"I'm sorry, but I think it's better to talk about it for a minute. I think it would be more appropriate for you to call him yourself. But if it's really important to you, of course I'll do it. It's up to you."

"No. It's up to you. I'm asking you to do it."

We stare at each other for a moment.

"Okay," I say. "I'll do it."

There's a pause. I take out a piece of paper.

"Can I get your number and your name, to give to them?"

"I already told you my name. But you don't have to remember everyone's name you hear."

His voice says the opposite of his words, and I sigh. There is nothing I can do about this at this point.

"I'm Jefferson," he says, finally.

"Okay," I say. "Jefferson—" He doesn't fill in the last name. I glance down at the patient sheet in front of me. "Harris."

I realize as soon as the name is out of my mouth that it's the wrong one, that the sheet in front of me is someone else's. Normally I wouldn't have made this mistake; normally I wouldn't have even had to look to come up with the name. But I was flustered and getting confused.

I know instantly that the mistake is a fatal one, and the knowledge is confirmed by the look of wide-eyed fury on the brother's face. "Harris? Who's Harris? That isn't even my fucking brother's name—"

"I'm sorry," I say, despair settling into the pit of my stomach. "I know. Your brother's name is Carson. Charles Carson."

He continues to stare.

"You're Jefferson Carson?"

"No," he says. "I'm Jefferson Williams. But I'm his brother."

"Okay," I say. "What's your number?"

He spells it out for me, then adds contemptuously, "If this is too complicated for you, just forget it."

Again, I think to myself, there's no point in fighting on this. I can't undo the mistake, can't recover the ground I've lost. I'd better just go on. "When will you be there?"

"What do you mean, when am I going to be there?"

I glance up. I wasn't trying to be difficult. "I was just asking when you thought you would be at home, when was the best time for them to call."

"I'll be there. I'll be there all the time until they call."

"You aren't there now; you're here. If you're going to be staying here for a while, I can have them call you here instead."

"I wouldn't have given you the number if I wasn't going to be there."

"Look," I say. "I'm only asking, because I'm trying to make it easier for them to reach you."

"Why don't you pay some attention to what's easier for *me* for once?"

I sit through another long pause, unable to come up with a response. "Fine," I say. "If there are no more questions? . . ." I glance briefly around the room. I nod at the girlfriend, the sisters, the brother, and walk out.

I go to the desk—walking by Mr. Carson's room on the way, "Oh, baby!"—and call the attending, who turns out to be in his office; easy enough to reach after all. I ask him to hold while I go get the brother, whom I lead to the phone without preamble.

Mr. Carson's note is the one thing I have left to do. I stand at the little desk outside his door, writing it. He's awake now, although when I went in he looked through and not at me, seemed unaware of my presence even while I examined him. "Ooh baby!" comes though the door. "Ooh baby, ooh baby—Woo!" I move, to finish my note elsewhere. If it's too painful for me to stand there and listen, what must his family be going through?

As I walk by the nurses' station on my way off the floor, I see the brother, still holding the phone, listening. Tears are streaming down his face.

I GO IN to check on Charles first thing the next morning. His brother is sitting at his bedside, holding his hand, brow deeply furrowed. Charles is still and quiet, his eyes closed.

I watch them for what feels like a long time. "How long have you known that your brother had cancer?" I ask at last.

"Three weeks," he says absently.

"I mean—" he adds. "I've known for months that there was something wrong, that he wasn't okay. A year maybe. But three weeks ago he found the strength to tell me."

I nod. I'm glad he heard the diagnosis from his brother and not from us.

MR. CARSON HAD decided earlier with his primary doctor that if his mind were to go, he would want to be allowed to die. Now his family, reluctantly, agrees that point has been reached. We back off on our level of medical support—not that there was much we could do for him anyway—and concentrate on keeping him comfortable.

I am on call that night. As it happens, I'm cross-covering on another patient who is dying and being kept on "comfort measures," a morphine drip and monitoring, nothing more to prolong life. Letting people die is not something we're as good at as keeping them alive. The nurses, uncomfortable with letting go, keep calling me.

"Mr. Carson's got a temperature. A hundred and two."

It's one in the morning, a nurse is on the phone.

"Oh," I say.

"Do you want me to do anything?"

"Is he uncomfortable?" I ask.

"No," she says. "But it's a fever. Can I give him Tylenol or something?"

How? I want to ask. He can't swallow anything. He can't have an NG tube, because he's got huge varices in his esophagus just begging to bleed at the least trauma. Do you want to roll him over and stick a suppository into his rectum to treat a fever he doesn't feel, disturbing a rest from which he isn't going to wake? Leave him alone.

"Look," I say. "He's comfort care. If he looks uncomfortable, we'll do everything we can to treat that. If he's not, then honestly, a fever is the least of his problems at the moment."

The silence on the phone manages somehow to sound wounded.

"So you're not going to do anything?"

"Not if he's not uncomfortable."

You're killing him, she says, without speaking the words.

I know, I answer by the same telepathy. And then—no. Cancer is killing him. I know he's young, I know it's tragic. But there is nothing you or I or anyone can do. We aren't giving up because we don't care; we're giving up because there's nothing left to do. I'm sorry. I'm sorrier than you can know—but it's not my fault.

MY PAGER RINGS again, an hour later, after the nursing change of shift. "It's Mr. Carson. He's wheezing a lot. I was wondering if we could

57

suction him out, drop a nasal trumpet down and try to get some of those secretions out of there?"

"He's a comfort care patient. He has a terminal disease and he's dying. We're not trying to prolong this."

"Oh," she says.

"Is he uncomfortable?"

"No."

"Then we'll leave him alone."

I will read the note in the chart in the morning. "Patient wheezing. Attempted to get permission to suction. Refused by Dr. Transue." The finger-pointing makes me sad and not a little guilty; "It's not my fault," I repeat, failing to soothe myself.

My pager goes off again a minute later. "About Mr. Eronton—" The other one, the cross-cover patient. I don't even know him, and I may be presiding over his death.

"Yes?" I take a deep breath.

"His heart rate bradied down into the forties. He's back up again now. I know we're not doing anything about it. We just have to let you know."

"Thank you," I say, sighing.

Another call. "On Mr. Eronton—"

"Yes?"

"They discontinued all his labs. But we've been giving him potassium replacement according to his lab each day. He usually needs about forty. Should I keep giving that, even without the labs, or just stop?"

It doesn't matter, I want to say. Don't you understand, it doesn't matter? He is *dying*.

Her voice says, she needs to do something. "Go ahead and give it to him," I say. It doesn't make any difference one way or the other. Perhaps this will make her feel better.

Every half hour all night long I get a call on the one or the other. But neither of them dies, that day or the next. I sign Mr. Carson out the following evening to cross-cover; "Just keep him comfortable. He may not last the night."

58

I go in to preround in the morning. I reach for Mr. Carson's chart in its compartment. It isn't there. I walk through the open door into his room, half expecting to find it empty, but it's not.

He lies in the bed, the blanket tucked in to his shoulders, quite still.

I can't decide for a moment if he's dead or only sleeping. I watch for movement under the sheets and see none. Then I notice the IV pump, the morphine drip, dangling forlornly in the corner. It's not connected. That means he's definitely dead.

I take a step closer to the bed. He doesn't really look dead, he just looks peaceful, after seeming so anguished for so long.

I peer at his face, trying to remember what he looked like when he first came in. It's a kind face, thoughtful, complicated; there is character there, depth.

I drift a little too close. Through his squinted lids I see the glazed, lifeless eyes, feel a sudden panic at being alone in a room with a corpse. Spinning, I grab my clipboard and rush out of the room.

Breathing heavily, I pick up one of my neighboring patient's charts and start flipping through it, to soothe myself. A nurse walks by. "Hey," I say. "Do you happen to know when Mr. Carson died?"

"Mr. Carson?"

I nod, gesture toward his room.

"Oh, I don't know," she says. "I've been out for a few days. I hadn't heard."

"No," I clarify. "He died last night. I didn't know what time. His body is still in there."

What language does one use, about this passage? "He's still in there" to imply, "He just happens to be dead, now." Or, "His body is still in there," suggesting that "he" left. I think about the words we use for death: deceased, expired, perished, passed on. We talk about demise, departure. So many subtle variations on the theme of leaving or ceasing to be or running out of time.

The nurse is staring at me. "What?"

I gesture toward the room.

"In there?"

I nod.

She glances around. "Does anybody know?"

"I think so," I say. "His IV was out."

"Usually they close the door, put a sign on it or something."

This relieves me, somehow. I'm glad you're not supposed to wander unknowing into rooms with dead bodies. She steps into the room, to check. I wonder if she doesn't trust me to declare a body dead. I am ever so slightly gratified when she comes bolting out again looking as spooked as I was. "I'll check with my supervisor," she says.

An hour later, as we go by on morning rounds, I see his family, clumped around his room, in the stooped postures of mourning. We have to pass them, to get to another of my patients. As we walk by, I glance the other way, afraid to look into his brother's face.

11. Dreaming

Internship envelops me in a way that I have never been enveloped by anything; medicine slips into my pores, permeates my conscious and unconscious worlds. From the beginning of the year, I have trouble sleeping, a particularly painful fact, given how little I am allowed to try. My dreams as well as my waking thoughts are saturated with medical content and anxiety. I dream cross-cover calls, codes, imaginary pages. As the year goes on I become more exhausted, less able to process or express, to myself or others, my experiences, fears, anxieties. I go numb on some level, and my days grow easier; but my nights become more haunted. What at first were tense but simple phantoms—imaginary patients created in rich detail, fantasy nursing calls for decreased urine output, chest pain, shortness of breath—give way to darker, more complex imaginings. I wake screaming in the night once, not knowing why. I fall asleep again at last, into strange, troubled dreams.

I find myself wandering through the hallways of a hospital that both is and isn't mine. Doors close and open. I drift in silence, seeking an uncertain destination. Then I am in a room standing over a patient, reaching down to take a pulse, when suddenly another stretcher is wheeled in, a crowd of people whirling around it. I turn as they transfer from the stretcher to the waiting bed the crumpled body of a young girl, maybe eleven or twelve, limp, clearly dead and not recently so, decomposing. I cannot smell the decay in the dream, but I remember thinking that I had to get out of the room or the smell would momentarily overwhelm me. I stand, stunned, and back out of the room. . . .

Then I am walking, hurriedly, back through the halls of the hospital, dark now, mostly empty. I pass through a door and into a commotion—angry faces, upset about what is happening upstairs, pushing, shoving. I turn back through the door, away from the mob. Then I proceed into a haunted game of hide-and-seek, trying to find a safe way out of the hospital, driven deeper and deeper into its dark depths. Suddenly there begin to be people again, angry people, faces twisted in fear and hatred. I step through the outside door, which I thought might be my last escape, but there they are again, the thronging masses, pulsing in fury.

I stand frozen, and from amidst them, rushing down the stairs which rise in front of me, comes a young mother, her head shrouded, carrying in her arms an infant—a strange infant, tiny, emaciated, and malformed, more like a strange plastic doll. She pushes the baby toward me. I reach out my hands to ward it off, find myself taking it instead. I can feel overwhelming pain and anger streaming from the child; it stares at me and speaks. "You didn't save her. You didn't try—"

"We tried," I answer, sadly and desperately—suddenly knowing more of the story, enough to know this. "We tried our best. We wanted to—but there are things that happen that we can't control, can't fix; there are times when everything we can do isn't enough. We failed, I failed, and I'm sorry—I'm so sorry—"

And suddenly I realize I am weeping, tears streaming abundantly down my face and bathing the child, until it is soaked in salt water. Its pale, plastic skin had seemed to burn before, but now, washed in tears, it cools. Suddenly the infant's anger is gone, it is calm and strangely whole. Though the baby doesn't speak, I am completely sure that it understands, has accepted my tears, and forgiven me. The cooling tears and the warmth of forgiveness wrap around me, and I breathe in the strange new air of peace.

12. Coffee

Ethel Lera was the only person I ever knew of who failed hospice. The definition of hospice is care in the last six months of life. It's always hard to know for sure, but people who are sent there generally have very little time left to them. Some outlive the six months, of course, but I'd never heard of anyone who took so long in dying that they finally gave up on it and went home.

Her primary physician told me the story the night she first came in. "She's got awful lungs," he said. "Pretty much the worst lungs you'll ever see on anyone who isn't dead. Four or five years ago, we sent her to a hospice facility. She'd been in the hospital every two or three weeks with terrible lung problems, intubated a bunch of times, more than I could count. Everyone agreed—even she agreed—it was enough. So off she went to hospice. Six months? I didn't think she'd last for one." He smiled. "Three years later they kicked her out. They said, Look, we're sorry, but we just can't keep you here any longer. They gave her a plaque when she left. She still has it, at home. I think they thought it was the only way they could get rid of her. They said she was the only person they'd ever had to send home."

Ethel Lera was a survivor. Furthermore, she was not someone who played by anyone else's rules, including modern medicine's.

SHE CAME IN very late one night, a thin, frail-looking old woman with wild white hair, accompanied by her earnest and worried primary care doctor, her daughter, and three of her grandchildren. She had a cough, a fever, had had some trouble breathing for the last few days. I tried to ask her questions, but she kept drowsing off midanswer. I had a distinct sense that she could have stayed awake if she liked, but that she was damned if she was going to let me disturb her rest. She'd squint at me as I shouted a question—she was quite deaf—ponder for a second, then close her eyes and mouth tightly, frowning.

"Her daughter can give you the whole story," said her doctor. "Let me just try with her for a second, though."

He bends close to her over the bed, and shouts in her ear.

"How much are you smoking, Ethel?" he asks.

She opens her eyes to squint at him. "I'm not," she answers, in the habitual yell of the hard of hearing.

He glances at her daughter. "A couple packs."

She turns to glare. Maybe she's not so hard of hearing after all? "No, you don't understand—" she begins.

"Understand what?"

"These new Basic cigarettes don't have any nicotine. Look at my fingers." She displays her clean hands proudly. "The Surgeon General won't even put a label on them—"

"*Ethel* . . ." He rolls his eyes at her. "You aren't falling for that marketing crap, are you?"

She hangs her head.

Smoking histories are measured in "pack-years"; one pack per day for one year is one pack-year. Ethel has amassed an astounding 280 pack-year smoking history. She's been smoking four packs of cigarettes a day for seventy years.

"She told me once she'd quit, only to break down the next visit and admit she'd lied," her doctor says.

"What's her code status?" I ask the attending quietly in the hallway after we've finished our interview. Would we put her on a ventilator if she reached a point where she couldn't breathe?

"Well . . ." he says, frowning—a bad beginning. "I've been over it with her, and she always says she wants everything done. I say, even tubes down your throat and pounding on your chest and electric shocks? And she says, Yeah, if you have to. But does she really know what that means? Her quality of life is pretty poor, her family's pretty tired, and so is she. I guess for the moment I can't say we wouldn't in-tubate. But don't transfer her to the ICU or anything, even if she gets sicker."

What I need to know is what I'm supposed to do if she suddenly goes downhill—try to save her, or let her go—and I'm not at all sure I've gotten an answer to that. But I nod slowly.

"She's likely to get worse before she gets better," he admonishes on his way out the door. "Just so you know—I really don't know if she'll make it through this."

THE NEXT MORNING she starts to decompensate. Early in the morning she looks all right. Then I get a call that her oxygen levels are dropping. I order a mask with more oxygen, and suctioning to clear the mucus out of her airways. They call back. It's helped a little, but not much. "Get a stat chest X-ray, and an ABG," I say. "I'll be up as soon as I can." I'm still rounding in the ICU when my pager goes off again. "Come now," says the nurse, the panic in her voice even more emphatic than her words.

"I'm on my way," I answer.

She looks awful. Breathing with great difficulty, her skin blue, her saturations dropping on the monitor. Shit.

I draw the blood gas, call the respiratory techs to get up here and readjust her high-oxygen mask. She's on the point of needing to be in-tubated. In spite of our discussion the night before, I still don't know whether or not to do that. "Don't transfer her to the ICU," her attend-ing had said. That means, don't intubate her. But did he really mean that if that was what she needed, I should let her die?

I call the attending's number. His secretary answers: "I'm sorry, he's not in this morning. I can take a message—"

"I need to talk to him now," I say.

"I think he's at his other office. I can give you that number."

Wanting to scream, I dial the second number. "He's not in just yet," a polite voice replies to my desperate request.

"Look," I say, starting to decompensate, myself. "I've got a patient of his here who's dying, he said he didn't want her tubed, but he never wrote an order not to, and *I don't know what the hell to do*, 'cause she's going to be dead in a couple minutes if I don't do anything, and *I need to talk to him right now, okay?*"

There's a moment's stunned pause on the other end of the phone. "I'll give you his home number," she says weakly.

"Thank you," I say.

The attending's young daughter answers the phone. It takes me a little while to persuade her to let me talk to Daddy. I'm close to crying by the time I get him on the line.

"She's crashing and I think she's about to need to be intubated—"

"Don't do that. Don't intubate her. Just try to hold things off until I can get there, okay?"

It's not that easy, I want to say. I can only hold off so long. And how can I not intubate her, if it comes to a choice between that and letting her die, since I don't have proof that either she or her family would prefer the latter?

But I let that go, pray it won't come to that. "The family isn't here," I tell him. "Someone needs to call them."

"Could you do it?" he asks. "Call her daughter. Tell her to come right in."

I dial the number. "This is Dr. Transue, from the hospital—"

"Yes," she says. "Of course."

"I don't want to alarm you, but I think it might be a good idea for you to come in—"

"I'm trying to," she says. "I have to get things set up for the baby-sitter, and lunches made for the older kids—I should be there in a few hours."

I try to figure out what to say next. I really don't know how to do this. How do you say, Don't panic, but I think your mother's dying?

"Unless . . ." she adds, realization dawning in the long silence on the phone.

"I think you should come as soon as possible," I say.

"I'll be right there," she answers.

BY THIS TIME we're using the most intense oxygen support that we have short of intubation: a mask that fastens over her mouth and nose, forcing pure oxygen into her airways. She still looks terrible, her skin bluish, her respirations labored, her oxygen still dropping.

She clutches at the mask, pulling it from her face. "Water—" she cries out hoarsely.

"Ethel . . ." I sigh. She's dying of hypoxia, and she wants to drink. "You need to concentrate on breathing right now. You can have a drink later."

"*Water*—" She sounds so pitiful, wrenching at my heartstrings, that I get a glass of water and go through great contortions to get her a sip between breaths, around the mask that covers her face.

I can see that she's still trying to mouth something. I pull the mask away to let her speak, and she gasps out a few words: "Where is my heart?"

At least, I think that's what she says; I can't tell for sure. I tap her chest; "Your heart is in here." She frowns, looking dissatisfied.

We put the mask back over her face—her oxygen level plummets instantly every time we take it away. "Try to write it out," I suggest, handing her a pen and my notepad.

She takes the pen, and scratches a strange series of careful squiggles with it. I can't read anything.

A nurse takes the pad from me. "I've spent a lot of time reading these; it's easy once you get the hang of it, you just have to trace their movements and imagine them along a straight line. See, like this."

She traces the letters, identifying them, and reads out from the squiggle:

"My heart is gone."

I stare at Ethel, trying to understand what this might mean. I can see her mouth moving again, frantically this time, through the clear plastic mask. She's trying to say something. I offer her the pad again, but she pushes it defiantly away.

Sighing, I lift the mask off her face for a moment, to let her speak.

She draws a deep breath.

"When can I go home?" she rasps.

She clutches tightly to my hand, and her huge blue eyes are desperate with entreaty.

"I'm not sure, sweetheart," I say, hearing my voice crack on the last syllable.

I release her hand, duck out of the room and dive for the bathroom. "Staff only," the door is marked, the local euphemism for staff lavatory— God forbid that we should share porcelain with the bottoms of the masses. But the bathroom is my respite, refuge, sanctuary. Here I may steal a moment alone, to breathe, to close my eyes, or to cry. I slump against the cool, reassuring solidity of the wall, let my fear and sadness overwhelm me for a minute.

AT LAST THE attending arrives. He agrees that the final decision point is near. He continues to believe we shouldn't put her on a ventilator.

"Look," he says. "I think we should not intubate on grounds of futility. I don't think she'd make it off the vent if we put her on. Her family agrees she's had enough, but they don't want to take responsibility for making the decision. I'm comfortable doing it, but we need another attending doctor to sign the papers."

At that moment, the pulmonologists appear, an attending and a fellow.

"This isn't futile," the fellow says, frowning. I will remember her later from this moment like a knight in shining armor at the door, championing the desperate cause. "Steroids and antibiotics might pull her through this, with a few days on the vent. There's a decent chance she'd leave the hospital. If she doesn't want to be tubed, that's one thing, but you couldn't call this futile."

They begin debating, and I become aware of my pager, which has gone off a dozen times in the last half hour. I suddenly remember that I'm supposed to be presenting a case at a conference that started five minutes ago.

"We'll take care of things," the attending says. "You go ahead."

I nod dumbly. "You'll call me if? . . ." I leave the question hanging.

He nods. "Of course."

I sit in conference, unable to concentrate. I stare at the paper she scribbled on, lying on top of my clipboard pile; I can read it now. "My heart is gone." I think to myself, the last words of a dying woman. What does it mean, what is she saying?

When I come back from conference, she's settled in the ICU, intubated, and lightly sedated. Sleeping, with the ventilator breathing for her, she looks peaceful, quiet, a picture of calm innocence.

AFTER THREE DAYS of aggressive treatment for infection and bronchospasm, her lung function improves, surprising us all, to the point at which we think she can breathe on her own. We extubate her on morning rounds, the entire team in the room as we deflate the small balloon which holds the tube in place and slide it out of her mouth.

She coughs, then takes a few raspy, experimental breaths. She surveys the room, stares from one to the next of us, studying us each long and carefully. Her big, blue eyes are wide and wild. Her hair, mussed by the tape that had protected the tube, springs around her face in a huge, chaotic halo.

She takes another long, deep scratchy breath. She's clearly about to say something. We all hold our breaths in anticipation. Will it be: "You should have let me die?" Or, "How could you have let things go so long?"

She takes one last, loud, endless breath.

"Coffee," she whispers, hoarsely.

There's a pause.

"Mrs. Lera," I say, "can I—"

"*Coffee!*"

I stare at her for a moment, nonplussed. She stares back at me. I shrug, turn to the nurse. "Get her some coffee. Decaf, please."

I COME BACK after rounds to check on her. She's had her coffee, and she studies me carefully as I walk in.

"Milk!"

"Excuse me?"

"Milk!"

"I'll have your nurse bring some milk in a minute. I just want to ask you a couple of questions, okay?"

"Who are you?"

"I'm Emily Transue. I'm one of the doctors taking care of you."

She wrinkles her nose. "How old are you?" she demands.

"Old enough," I say, smiling.

"You're a Dougie Howser," she says.

"How old are you?" I ask.

"Too old," she answers immediately.

Hm. I'm trying to get a sense of how well oriented she is, but she's not helping. "Can you tell me your full name?"

She stiffens. "I'm Ethel Williams Lera, I live at twenty-five Andrews Place, Seattle, nine-eight-one-zero-four. The year is 1974, the date is July fifteenth," she announces, in a loud, clear voice, finishing with flourish.

She stares at me defiantly. I choke back a smile. She got the name right, anyway, but it's all in the presentation.

"I'm leaving," she says.

"Excuse me?" Why do I keep saying that?

"I'm going home. I don't want to be here anymore. The food is bad. I want to go home."

"Mrs. Lera, a few days ago you almost died because you couldn't breathe. You're doing better now, but I still think—"

"I want my daughter!" she yells, cutting me off.

I look around.

"She left," the nurse says, with a little roll of her eyes as much as to say, You couldn't really blame her.

"You can't keep me here! I want to talk to my daughter!"

The nurse looks up. "She's been like this all day. We have her daughter's number—"

I shrug, and the nurse dials the phone. As I walk out of the room, I hear her speaking loudly and deliberately into the receiver:

"I'm in the hospital, I'm raising hell, I want to go home."

GIVEN HOW SICK she was, the speed of her recovery is almost miraculous. Antibiotics and steroids work their magic, and within forty-eight hours she's out of the ICU. We start making tentative discharge plans.

"Hey, Mrs. Lera," I say, the morning after she's transferred to the floor.

"Hey, Dougie Howser." She's settled into the nickname, to my distress.

"How do you feel?"

"With my hands." She doesn't miss a beat. "I'm going to go home," she says.

"Yes," I say, "I know. Maybe even tomorrow."

"*Today*. I'm going today."

"Okay," I say. "Maybe today."

She rolls her eyes at the silly young doctor who hasn't figured out yet that once she decides she wants something, she's going to get it.

I change the subject. "Are you going to quit smoking?"

"Sure."

"I don't think I believe you."

She doesn't answer. I shake my head.

"I'm glad you're better," I say suddenly. I look at her fondly, and something in my eyes must strike her, because she reaches out and clasps my arm tightly for a moment. Then she lets go and turns away, sighing.

I talk to the attending and, with his approval, write her discharge orders. She will indeed go home today.

13. Connection

I'm sitting at a desk in the ICU, writing notes on the two patients whose rooms are on either side of me. It's a familiar ritual. Other patients come and go, but these two have been here almost two months each, both on ventilators most of the time, both teetering endlessly on the edge of death. I am a fixture in the ICU for a few hours each morning, hovering between the two, conferring with their consultants, writing notes and orders.

My pen slows to a halt, and I find my thoughts drifting. I consider the two of them, their charts splayed out before me on the desk. They're both terribly ill, almost hopeless. I've poured countless hours of thought and work into each. Yet I feel very differently about the two. One of them I sweat blood and tears for, lie awake at night worrying about. The other, the one whose note I'm writing now, is just another piece of work, another responsibility. I try equally hard to take good care of him, but the emotional content is completely different. My heart just isn't in it. His wife, I care about his wife—plump, powdered, insistently cheerful and upbeat, always fussing about me and whether I'm getting enough sleep. I worry about her endless denial of his illness, her refusal to budge from the caretaking role. But I just don't have that connection to her husband.

How does this happen? The chemistry that happens between doctors and patients, the natural sympathy that is so strong in some interactions and so elusive in others, I sensed intuitively when I first started clinical work, but began to try to analyze only later. I have come to think that doctors and patients, like lovers or friends, can have a deep instinct to connect with each other in some instances and not in others. You can work around the connection, care for someone without it, learn to modulate it; the bond can appear suddenly after a long time of being absent. But that basic chemistry is real.

Why, I wonder, should that be so dramatically different for these two men, when neither of them has ever really even been able to talk to me?

Maybe it's because one of them seems to be fighting—fighting us, sometimes, as actively as his illness. How many lines have I replaced that he's pulled out, in rage or confusion, while the other just lies there, passive in the face of disease and intervention. We spent weeks struggling to wean him from the ventilator, and finally succeeded. When the tube was removed from his throat, unlike most patients who quickly return to rather hoarse and breathless speech, he stayed silent, rousing himself to whisper only the rare word. Usually after someone is extubated, his room becomes suddenly more alive with noise, movement. With him, the only change seemed to be the absence of the breathing machine and its loud, mechanical sighs.

Maybe I'm wrong. Maybe it was nothing that he did or didn't do that caused my apathy. Perhaps I couldn't afford to care. Perhaps there are limits to how much a person has to give, and I had simply reached mine.

Whatever the cause, in spite of all that time and work, we'd never bonded. I cared for him with my mind, but not my heart. Was that so wrong? It came to the same thing medically, and it was easier on me. Sighing, I stop philosophizing and return to writing his note.

A FEW DAYS later, I go into his room for my daily morning check.

"How are you feeling?" I ask, in my usual tone of exaggerated brightness.

He, as usual, doesn't answer.

"Are you breathing okay?"

He nods.

"Do you have pain anywhere?"

"No," he manages to whisper.

I ask a few more simple questions, then go on to my exam. Neck, heart, lungs, abdomen, then a brief neuro check. He lies limply while I tap out his reflexes. "Wiggle your toes." He obliges, one foot and then the other.

I take his left hand. "Squeeze my hand." There is a slight but definite pressure from his fingers.

"Great!" Sometimes he's not able to do this.

"Now squeeze my other hand."

Again the pressure. "Terrific!" I'm not even sure how much of my enthusiasm is real and how much feigned.

He releases my hand slowly. I am bent over him, and he looks up at me thoughtfully. His expression is somehow different from usual.

"What is it?" I ask.

He draws a breath as if about to say something. He beckons with a twitch of one finger, and I lean closer, listening for his whisper.

With a heavy, shaking hand he reaches slowly across the few inches which separate us and brushes his fingers, ever so lightly, across my cheek. His hand stays suspended there, barely touching my face, for a long moment. Then he drops his hand to his lap, smiles mysteriously, and closes his eyes.

I stare at him for a long moment. His smile does not fade, but he does not open his eyes.

Strangely shaken, I go on to my other work, recognizing that something irreversible has just happened. He just crossed the invisible line from being a patient to being a person. For better or worse, we're connected now.

THE CHANGE AFTER that is subtle. He never does anything like that again. He doesn't become more active or involved really, but I think there's a certain light in his eyes that wasn't there before. And I know that neither the gentleness nor the enthusiasm in my voice when I talk to him is faked.

A few days later, I go off service. On my last day, I sit on his bed, take his hand, and tell him that someone else will come to take my place. He doesn't really react. I have a week's vacation. I leave town, and the moment I come back, I rush to visit him. I walk into his room, where nothing seems to have moved or changed since I left the week before. I take his hand. His eyes look through me, unseeing, and he gives no sign of recognition.

"It's like he just gave up," his new intern tells me, calling a week later to tell me that he'd died. "I don't know what he was like when you were there, but from the time I came on—it was like he'd just decided it was time to die. And he did.

"It's sad . . ." he finishes uncertainly.

"Yes," I say. "It is."

14. Nightclub

The music is loud, the lights are dim. The crowd on the dance floor is packed and swaying.

It's later than I should be out. I have to work early tomorrow, as I always do. I'm sipping a beer, although I don't really like beer, and—pushing the same illogic even further—I'm sharing puffs of my friend's cigarette, although I don't smoke. Something about this evening calls for contradictions.

I'm here with my friend and fellow intern Chris, but we aren't dancing. We're sitting with our beers on the black counter that runs along the perimeter of the club. We sit in silence for a while, mesmerized, immersing ourselves in the loud pulsing music, the young, healthy bodies swirling on the dance floor. Everything seems so simple here. For a moment it feels as if we could drown the complexities of our lives in that primal, mindless beat.

I WOULD BE hard-pressed to explain what I'm doing here, what brings me to a smoky, loud, meat-market nightclub at one o'clock on a Thursday morning, five hours before I have to be at work. I suppose I'm here because I'm twenty-five years old and the most rebellious thing I will have done with my twenty-sixth year, besides sharing a half dozen cigarettes, will be to call in sick for exactly one half day of clinic to go skiing. Because

I'll feel guilty about that half-day. Because most nights that I'm not in the hospital I'm in bed asleep by ten, and most evenings that I have energy to do anything I spend at the gym, trying to prevent this life I have chosen from stealing my physical strength as it has stolen so much else.

But this is more than just rebellion. I'm here because sometimes— overwhelmed by exhaustion, stress, the constant weight of responsibilities I don't know how to handle, the ever-present, insatiable demands of other people's needs and emotions—I get so numb that I can't even remember what it would be like to feel. The music that is pulsing in my bones, my skin, my chest, reminds me. The drums seem almost to remind my weary heart to beat. I've gotten so used to being the observer that once in a while I need to be a participant—though look at me, even now: not dancing, just watching. Still, the music is for me as much as for anyone. I am not a doctor here, I am anonymous, insignificant.

I fill my lungs with the thick dark air, saturated with smoke and sweat and hormones. There's flesh, skin, everywhere; all I see are naked arms, the occasional bare muscled chest, and eyes, eyes seeking and finding, chasing and running away, edged glances sharp with meaning. The room pulsates, a living thing. I wrap myself in it, this dark, wild profusion of life. At this moment, I can admire youth in its fatal imagined immortality, its pure naive stupidity, the largesse with which it squanders and throws itself away.

Chris turns to me, and yells over the noise: "Do you really want to be a doctor for the rest of your life?"

Laughing—at his choice of topic, at the similarity of his thought processes to mine—I answer. "I don't even want to be a doctor for the rest of the week, especially."

But he says, "No, I'm serious. What are you going to do with the rest of your life?"

I sigh. "That's hard. I don't see myself in private practice. Maybe academe . . ." Are we really having this conversation here?

"Do you ever think," he says, "that academe is just an out for people who aren't sure they like medicine? I mean, don't like it enough to just do that for the rest of their lives?"

"Maybe," I say. "Yes, maybe."

I think for a minute.

"What do you want?" I ask him. "In your life."

"I don't know," he says.

A pause.

"It's just so hard—"

We study the crowd for a while.

"Do you think it gets easier?" I ask.

"Which part?"

"All of it." I think for a minute. "Like: do you think there will come a time when I'm not scared—panicked—the way it seems I am most of the time when I'm working, now?"

He pauses.

"Most of the time?" he asks.

I shake my head, jump off the counter, extend a hand to him. It's too loud to talk, and we talk enough as it is. It's time to dance.

15. Raspberry Strudel

"Fuck."

I turn, startled, to face my resident, who has just spoken. It is through his voice that I hear it, tune my ears to listen to the loud-speaker I was tuning out before; "Code one ninety-nine," it repeats. "Room two fifty-five C."

We stare at each other for an instant, then around, momentarily disoriented. Which way?

"There . . ." A helpful nurse pushes me in the right direction. She hears the call but her job is to stay behind. I break into a run.

It's a room in the Cardiac Care Unit. The man is in his sixties, a day or two post-op from a coronary bypass. The cardiac surgeon appears fast on our heels, his mouth tight, his brow furrowed in a deep frown.

He looks partly upset and partly angry. This was not supposed to happen, his expression clearly says.

Will it hurt your numbers, your percentages? I wonder unkindly.

The patient is already fully monitored, clearly in arrest. Sudden cardiac death, ventricular fibrillation, presumably resulting from some combination of his coronary artery disease and the surgery designed to fix it. The surgeon takes charge of the code—I'm used to residents running codes, but perhaps the cardiac surgeons do their own—and the rest of us shift into a supporting role, carrying out orders.

I step into position and start chest compressions. I look down at the patient, a big man, his skin pale and flabby and bluish. The surgical scar down the middle his sternum is unhealed. It wriggles slowly open as the minutes pass, under the stress of my compressions; his blood oozes out, reddening in the oxygenated air. I feel the slipperiness of the blood beneath my gloves.

I am aware of a large unhealed wound on my palm where I scraped my hands on the pavement after tripping a few days ago. I feel the scab softening, loosening under the wet heat of my sweat inside my gloves. I feel the glove sliding, between the slipperiness of sweat on my side and blood on his, bunching up off my wrist, leaving my palm uncovered. I have an image of blood mingling with blood, yet my hands mechanically continue pumping.

IMAGINE WHEN BLOOD was only blood, how simple life must have been back then. Imagine the days when students on their first day of medical school drew blood—as we did, too—but instead of saving the tubes for future analysis as we did, they poured them all together into a bowl and each of them drank. Revolting, certainly, yet powerful.

Simple, I say, but maybe I really mean complicated. Imagine when blood was allowed to be a symbol, a bond, a connection, a culling of essence. Imagine when blood was about fear and fire and love and history—

And now blood means only viruses. Cold and clinical, decisive, divisive.

I'M BECOMING TIRED and someone touches my shoulder, steps in to relieve me. I strip off my bloody, sweaty gloves, scrub my hands for a moment at the sink, not certain if it is worse to open my cuts further. I put on a new pair of gloves and step back to the bedside, glancing at the patient, then focusing on the monitor. Funny how the screen and not the bed is where the locus of decision making lies. What to do next, whether to shock or no, and what medications to give, depends more on the electrical signals picked up by the chest leads than on anything you can hear or feel. With someone to relay basic exam information, you can run a code from afar with just the monitor. The residents in the ER do this all the time, running codes in ambulances on their way in. The monitor tracings are transmitted automatically to a special room in the ER, the ambulance staff radios information like the blood pressure and whether they can feel a pulse, and the doctor radios back to them what to do. I haven't had to do this yet, I can't imagine how it will feel: the disembodied clinical detachment of a code carried to its bizarre final extreme. Yet the patient seems irrelevant to what's happening in this room, even now.

MY TURN AGAIN in the CPR cycle. His rib cage has very little give to it, it's hard to do good compressions.

"You can get better leverage if you hop onto the bed," someone says.

He's bleeding, out of his mouth where the tube was put down, out of the site in his neck where the thick IV enters his body, snaking toward his heart. As I clamber up onto the bed and settle into a good position to do compressions—one knee above his shoulder, the other at his side—I am kneeling in a pool of blood.

The next time, relieving my replacement, I grab a towel and drop it on the bed below me. "Better traction," I say, to no one in particular, apparently feeling a need to explain away my discomfort.

I continue my rhythmic pushing, looking down at his chest sometimes, up at the monitor often, critiquing my compressions as they show up on the screen, trying to keep them strong and steady. I look around at the other faces, the nurses, my resident, the respiratory techs. Some look scared, some bored, some unsure what to do. A social worker who isn't involved stands there, wide-eyed and fixed on the spot, staring. I wonder what she was doing when all this began, what's going on inside her head. Then there is the surgeon, his face flat and unreadable, maintaining control.

My eyes settle on the curtain, half-closed against the curious passersby in the hallway, the frightened families of other, more fortunate patients. Then on the wall, the window. It's dark in the room, the window is too bright for me to focus on anything outside. I am hot, and weary. And I feel nothing, nothing for the big blue man beneath my fists.

And then I suddenly smell strudel. Raspberry strudel, clear as day there in that room of blood and death. I dismiss it as a fleeting hallucination, but it persists. Maybe someone in the room—the nurse across the bed from me, whom I lean toward as I bend over him—is wearing raspberry perfume, or raspberry lip gloss, and the smell is translating into strudel. That must be it. Either that or my brain is embarking on a bizarre, forced sensory escape.

"How long are we going to do this?" someone murmurs. It's been almost an hour, without any hopeful signs.

"Give it ten more minutes," the surgeon says. In his voice is the awareness that he's being unreasonable, that it's time to call it; but a plea also, for just a little more time.

The minutes tick slowly on the wall clock. I wonder if that's why they have clocks in every room—for timing codes—before realizing that's ridiculous.

"How many doses of Epi have we given?" the surgeon asks. "Let's give one more."

"Your ten minutes are more than up," a nurse points out, smiling to soften her implication.

"Give it a little longer."

Damn, I think. Enough. I'm tired. People stand ready to relieve me but somehow, at this point, I want to continue to the end. I can see my compressions traced on the monitor. I force myself to keep them strong.

"Okay," he says at last. "Enough."

And this time I am the one who pulls off bloodied gloves, washes my hands carefully at the sink, then grabs my coat to scramble away. A man is dead. I don't know who he was. I don't even know his name.

I remember hearing, murmured in the background of the code, that his wife had been called, that she was on her way in. I don't want to see her, I don't want to know.

"They have clean scrubs in the OR," my resident points out, glancing at my bloodied knees.

I nod. But I get stopped on the way back through the ICU, other patients, other responsibilities. The blood dries and I forget it. So I spend the rest of the day with his blood on my trousers, this nameless dead man. Late that night, I glance at the brown patches on my pants, as if I could glean something about him from that bit of fluid that oozed out of his body.

But all I see is pigment, nothing more.

16. Valencia

I was angry about Mr. Stone before I even met him.

He had come in to the hospital the day before with a massive pulmonary embolism. He collapsed at his son's house and was brought in by the medics. A spiral CT of his chest showed a saddle embolism—a huge blood clot lodged in his pulmonary artery, cutting off blood flow to both his lungs. He was given thrombolytics, powerful clot-dissolving drugs that were developed for treating heart attacks and are experimental in pulmonary embolism. His response was near miraculous. The clot dissolved, his blood pressure and oxygen levels rose, he woke up.

He was moved to the step-down unit, a kind of halfway point between ICU care and the regular ward. Now the ICU team wants to transfer him to my team, the ward team. My resident argues briefly with the ICU resident—he doesn't sound stable, he's still got very abnormal labs and unsteady vitals, shouldn't they watch him for another day?—then gives in and accepts the transfer. All morning, busy with other work, I get called every fifteen minutes, because his pressure is low or his oxygen is dropping or his electrolytes are off. I haven't even had time to talk to him yet, much less review his chart. I'm fuming at the ICU team for doing this to me, at my resident for accepting it, at the system for creating this kind of situation.

All this melts away the moment I walk into his room. He's a small man, dwarfed by the big hospital bed. He has huge gray-blue eyes, round and gentle, a thoughtful face, and a winning smile. He's extremely thin. The combination of his slender paleness, his gentle eyes and smile, and his flowing white beard give him a beatific appearance. I feel as if I should kneel and kiss his rings, or perhaps reach out to polish his halo.

His voice is faint and hoarse. He says it's been this way for a while, he's not sure how long, though it got worse after he was intubated for the pulmonary embolus. I find myself holding very still and leaning close to hear his words. But we get by.

I go over his history, which is fairly simple. He was healthy until a few weeks ago, when he was hospitalized elsewhere for a pneumonia that turned out to be caused by nocardia, an unusual infection, generally seen in people who are already sick or immunosuppressed in some way. He was quite sick initially, but improved quickly and was able to go home to his son's house. He doesn't live around here, he explains, he was visiting his son when all this happened. He was getting better, then he collapsed, but he doesn't remember anything more until he woke up here.

I ask if he's noticed any other symptoms lately, weight loss, fevers, cough, and so on. He says he's lost a little weight, he's not sure how much, and hasn't noticed anything else. He's always had a smoker's cough, despite giving up cigarettes five years ago, but it's no worse now. He felt fine until he got the pneumonia a few weeks ago.

When I examine him, I notice the enormous lymph nodes in his neck. The ICU team had mentioned these. The limited CT that diagnosed his pulmonary embolus also showed large nodes in his chest. A repeat chest CT was being done that morning to evaluate more closely.

We review the CT later in the day in X-ray rounds. As the film appears on the board, my heart sinks. Even I can pick out the huge lymph nodes in his chest, converging in his mediastinum to form a mass.

"Any chance that that could be reactive, from his nocardia infection?" my resident asks.

The radiologist shakes his head. "Tumor, tumor, tumor," he says.

It all fits together. The recent infection with an unusual organism, suggesting immunosuppression, the pulmonary embolus, suggesting a hypercoagulable state. His extreme thinness. His age, and his history of smoking. Everything points to cancer.

But how do we proceed? We need to make a definitive diagnosis, which means doing a biopsy; but I'm not certain of what. My resident tells me to talk to the Pulmonary person. I call her and go over the details of the case.

"So what's your question?" After a second she answers herself. "What do we do next?"

"That's the question," I agree.

"I think the best idea is to biopsy those nodes in his neck. It's a lot easier than going in for something in his lungs, and it will almost certainly give us a tissue diagnosis."

"That's what I thought," I say.

"So give the general surgeons a call. Ask them to come by."

I page General Surgery, sketch the story for them. "This is a sixty-nine-year-old man, former smoker, admitted with a large pulmonary embolus. He got thrombolytics, did really well as far as the embolus goes. However, he's got huge nodes in his neck, and a mass in his mediastinum by CT. We're very concerned for malignancy. We wondered if you'd take one of the nodes out of his neck."

"Why?" the surgeon asks. I've never liked this particular surgeon.

"So we can get a tissue diagnosis."

"Why not go in for something from his lungs?"

"Because the neck nodes are very close to the surface, a lot easier to get at than getting lung tissue, even by bronchoscopy."

"That's odd."

I'm not sure what's so odd about it, so I don't say anything.

"Tell me more about him."

"He's been pretty healthy, until a recent admission for nocardia—"

"So the nodes could be just from the infection." His voice is challenging, even dismissive.

"Could be. But he's got the mass in his mediastinum. The radiologists were pretty definite that it didn't look reactive, it looked like tumor."

"So the radiologists thought they could make a diagnosis?" The contempt in his tone is even thicker now.

"They felt the appearance was much more consistent with tumor than infection," I say with all the calm and professional manner I can muster.

"That's odd."

I decide not to answer.

"Well, okay then," he concedes, after a long pause. "We'll come have a look at him."

"Yeah, fuck you," I murmur to the air as I hang up the phone.

I'M EATING DINNER in the basement cafeteria a few hours later when his nurse pages me. "I was just curious—what . . . do you think is going on with him?"

"Well," I say, "we're pretty worried that he's got lung cancer."

"Oh," she says, in the tone of someone absorbing something expected but nonetheless difficult. "I wondered about his hoarseness. He says it's been that way for a while, since before he came in. But I thought it might be just from being intubated, for that little while with the PE."

"It might be," I say. "But his being hoarse isn't the only reason we're thinking about malignancy. He's got huge lymph nodes, and his CT shows a chest mass."

"Really?" She sounds startled. "The one they did this morning?"

"Yes."

"Oh . . ." Her voice is pained. I wish I could comfort her, but I don't know how.

"The surgeons are going to come see him," I go on, "about biopsying one of those nodes in his neck. Then we'll know for sure. But the radiologists were pretty sure it would be tumor. Small-cell lung cancer maybe, but it's hard to say. We'll see what the tissue shows first. The surgeons should be by tonight."

"Does he know that?"

It hits me like a ton of bricks that he doesn't, that I should have told him—about all of this, not just the biopsy. Somehow in the rush of everything I've been trying to do today, I didn't even think of it. Any moment now the surgeons are going to be marching in, not knowing what he does and doesn't know, saying who knows what. I cringe at the possibilities that flash suddenly through my mind. "So we're going to take this node out of your neck and find out what kind of cancer you've got. . . ." I do not know what to do, what to say to him, but I have a sinking certainty that I need to talk to him before they do.

My heart in my throat, filled with a sudden terrible urgency, I hang up the phone, leaving my half-eaten dinner on the table, and race toward his room. Breathless with seven flights of stairs, I find myself a few minutes later at his door. His light is out, but he's awake. He looks at me with wide eyes.

"Hey," I say softly.

"Hello."

I clear my throat, at a loss for words. I realize that I haven't figured out at all what I'm going to say, how I'm going to do this. I should have stopped, at least for a few minutes on the way up here, to think, but it's too late now. He watches me expectantly.

"I just wanted to let you know . . ." I begin. "We're going to have a surgeon come in to talk to you."

He gives me a questioning look. I sit down heavily on the side of his bed, trying to think how to go on. How could I have done this, how could I have walked in here so unprepared?

"Have you noticed the lymph nodes in your neck?" I ask at last. "You've got little lumps, along your neck—those are lymph nodes. Everyone has them, but they aren't usually that big. Have you felt them?"

"Sometimes," he says.

I continue. "The scan that we did this morning shows that you've got some big nodes in your chest, too. We're not sure why those are there. We want to take one of the nodes out of your neck, so we can look at it under the microscope and find out for sure what it is."

He nods. After finding brief comfort in the flow of words, of process, I'm left silent before the question in his eyes. I can't leave it there, I realize. I have to go on.

"It could be a couple of different things," I say. "For instance—the nocardia. The infection you had in your lungs? An infection like that can cause your nodes to get big."

He nods. That's not enough, a voice says gently in my head. It's easier for me to not say the rest, but I owe it to him to finish. I have to acknowledge his fears, and the truth. I glance down at the floor, trying to find words. Then I force myself to meet his eyes.

"Or it could be something more serious," I say slowly. "For example, there's a possibility it could be cancer."

There it is, the critical word, finally out, hanging in the air. He nods slowly, as if he had been waiting for this all along, which he probably has. He's probably guessed this on some level, just as I am sure of it on another level, though we are both clinging to the remaining uncertainty.

"We need to know," he says softly.

I watch him, powerless, for a moment.

"I know this is impossible to do, but if you can, try not to worry," I say. "We don't know anything yet. The biopsy will tell us, one way or the other. It might not be. We just don't know."

He nods, but I can see that his eyes are focused somewhere far away, that he's no longer listening.

"I don't want you to panic," I repeat. "I just wanted to let you know that the surgeons would be coming—so it wouldn't be a surprise."

"Thank you," he says quietly. "It's kind of a shock."

There's another pause, as I try to find something I can say. Something, anything, to ease or at least acknowledge the pain of this moment. But words fail me. I reach out to take his hand, and he clasps mine tightly.

"I'm sorry to be the one to tell you. . . ."

"You did a good job," he says. He smiles at me, his wide eyes sad and kind.

"I'm sorry," I say again.

"It's okay," he says.

We sit there, holding each other's hands, for a long time. My pager buzzes, once and then again, at my side. I ignore it. "Do you have any questions?" I ask finally.

"No," he says.

I pause. "If you think of anything, they can always reach me."

He murmurs something I can't hear at first. I lean closer.

"What's to ask?" he says with a wry smile.

My heart feels close to breaking as I return his wistful look.

"I TOLD HIM that it could be cancer," I say to his nurse, on the way out. "Just so you know he knows."

She nods. "We'll talk more about it later."

She frowns, suddenly. "He's lost forty pounds in a few months, he told me."

I nod. I remember how he refused to estimate a number for me earlier.

"He looks bad," she says. "He looks like somebody who's got something bad."

LATE THAT NIGHT, I am pacing the hospital, searching for something, some kind of comfort or peace which eludes me. I finish my work, find myself with a precious free moment, don't know what to do. The image of his face haunts me.

I find myself back at his door, unsure why I am there, but at the same time quite certain that it is the only place for me to be, my only chance at finding whatever I'm looking for. He is awake, watching television.

"I came to check on you."

"That's nice of you. Thank you."

He turns down the volume on the television.

"What are you watching?" The instinct telling me to come here wasn't accompanied by one telling me what I should say.

"A documentary on Thomas Jefferson."

"Is it good?"

He nods.

There's a long silence, which feels awkward but somehow more right than chitchat.

"Is there anything we can do for you?" I ask at last, tentatively. The "we" sounds strange, false, coming off my tongue. We've gotten beyond the impersonal hospital "we" which I sometimes represent. I'm here as myself, not as a system.

"Send me home," he says.

I sigh. "I'm afraid that's not a good idea yet. You aren't stable enough to be home now. But we'll send you home as soon as it's safe to."

He nods, actually smiles at this.

Slowly the silence becomes more comfortable. We talk a little, softly, in the half darkness. A nurse comes in to draw labs on his roommate.

"It's strange, having a roommate," he murmurs. "It's been a long time since I had such a thing."

"Do you live alone?" I ask. Normally I would have asked all this when he was admitted, but you miss things sometimes with patients who came in to another team.

He thinks for a minute. "That's a tough question."

I raise my eyebrows.

"I have—a companion. Who stays with me sometimes. But normally I live alone."

I nod. "It's good to have a companion."

"Yes." He nods seriously.

"Lucky companion." I smile at him.

"Lucky me." He smiles back.

There's another pause. "Is it true that you used to live in Spain, in Valencia?" I ask, looking for a conversation topic, and remembering a cryptic note in his chart which I'd meant to ask about further.

"Yes. Well—I still do, in a way."

"How did that happen?"

"I moved there, for a few years, long ago. After I was divorced. And then I've lived there since I retired. I think of it as home now. Bella, my companion, lives near there also."

"I see."

"But I have lots of friends in Seattle, too. Former colleagues. I used to work at Seattle University. . . ."

"What did you do?"

"Romance and Renaissance studies."

I nod. "My mother is an English professor—Victorian lit. That's where she started, now she mostly does women's studies. In Toledo, Ohio."

"That's wonderful!" His eyes light up, and he nods.

"When did you retire?"

"Five years ago. When I was sixty-four.

"I was very lucky," he adds absently. I'm not sure if he means lucky for retiring, or for working that long. I don't ask and he doesn't explain.

"You should sleep," I say after we've talked a while longer.

He nods. "I'm afraid I'll have trouble sleeping."

"We can give you something, to help," I say. Such an easy thing! Something I can do to make him feel better.

"Maybe that would be a good idea," he says slowly.

"We'll try it," I say.

"Thank you for coming," he says. "You've—made it better."

I don't ask what he means by "it." "I've enjoyed talking with you." I smile, and squeeze his hand.

He smiles, his startling wonderful grin shining after me as I walk out of the room.

"I'm writing him for a sleeper," I inform his nurse.

"Oh—great!" she says. "He thought it might be hard to sleep. He's—anxious. About everything."

"I would be, too," I say.

"We talked about it," she says. "After the surgery people came. He said, 'They're going to take out one of my lymph nodes.'

"I said, 'Do you know why they're doing that?'

"He said, 'Yes. They're afraid I have cancer.' "

She looks up. "Then he told me, he's been terrified he had cancer for five years."

I think to myself: ever since he retired . . .

She goes on. "Then he says: 'I don't have it. I don't have cancer. . . .' He was very definite." She shrugs kindly. "He's reacting very normally, very appropriately."

I nod. "Denial has its place."

I feel less hurt, less vulnerable after seeing him, knowing that he's okay. So often, trying to envision things through my patients' eyes, I simply can't imagine how they cope. I think that if someone gave me the news that I give them, I would simply perish, explode, cease to exist. I cannot imagine how my chronic pain patients live with their pain, how my sexual abuse survivors live with their memories, how my mentally ill patients can navigate their chaotic, shifting worlds. I don't know how someone gets through the first night of knowing they're going to die. But I'm endlessly amazed to discover, over and over, the strength that people have; their ability to muster coping mechanisms, their ways of managing and going on, surviving the moment, surviving the night.

By morning Mr. Stone has become almost businesslike about his not-yet-established diagnosis.

"I need to figure out how much time I have," he says. "There are things I have to do." He looks up at me gravely. "I've been commissioned to make a teapot."

"Really?" I say.

"I've taken up pottery since I retired. I have a wheel in Valencia, and there's a nearby oven which lets me fire things. There's quite a little demand for my services among my acquaintances." He catches my eye, to make sure I am taking this seriously. "And a very dear friend has commissioned a teapot. They are my specialty. . . ." He smiles demurely, then gives a serious nod. "I promised."

"Okay," I say.

He pauses, lost in thought for a moment.

"I can't complain. I've done what I set out to do in life."

"We'll—we'll try to help you do whatever is left on your agenda."

He likes this phrasing. He grins. "You're splendid," he says suddenly and warmly.

THE BIOPSY RESULTS come back two days later, confirming small-cell lung cancer. This time my resident comes with me to tell him. We walk in together, and I sit on the edge of his bed. He looks up at me and says, "You must be here about the lymph node results."

I nod.

"Well?"

"The biopsy shows that you have lung cancer."

He nods slowly, looks away briefly, then looks up at me. "We knew that, really, didn't we?"

I nod. "I'm sorry—" I clasp his hand.

He squeezes mine back. "It's okay." He shakes his head, then smiles a little, resigned smile. "Truly, it's okay."

A FEW DAYS pass, as he continues to stabilize, his system recovering from the pulmonary embolus, his blood pressure and respiratory function returning to normal.

He tells me about Valencia. He describes the twisting cobbled streets to me, the blueness of the sky, the gardens, the graceful stone houses. He tells me how he fell in love with it when he went there long ago, how he vowed to go back, and finally did. He tells me how it's changed over the years, but how the essence of it feels somehow the same, feels

90

as if it had been the same for centuries. As he talks his eyes are at once wistful and sweet with tenderness.

He tells me about Bella, his companion, also.

"Does she know?" I ask.

"No," he says. "Not yet."

"Do you want us to help you call her?" I ask. We know now that his hoarseness is from the tumor invading the nerves to his larynx. His voice is not going to get better. He's learned to speak in a very intelligible whisper, but it doesn't transmit well on the phone.

"She doesn't have a telephone," he says. "She lives on a little island where there are no phones. I will have to write to her. But I've contacted another friend, who will be able to go to see her and tell her."

I nod.

"I worry, about how she will react," he says. "She's—she's very brave." He pauses. "She has a lot of trouble with her nerves—but in another way she's very brave."

I nod.

For the rest of the day, walking through the hospital with its white walls and sterile hallways, I am beset with images of a different world—a world of islands without telephones, of sunshine on blue water and rose-colored bricks, narrow paths of stones through wild curving gardens. Chained as I am to my pager, confined to the narrow angled white passageways, I am almost unable to imagine that there could be a world like that out there. But I cling to my fantasy Valencia like a drowning person to a raft.

EVERY TIME I see him, I ask if there's anything he needs, anything I can do to make things better. Generally he shakes his head, and smiles. One day he pauses after the question, looking uncertain.

"What is it?" I ask.

"Well . . . I wondered if perhaps—" He breaks off. "My neighbor here left," he says, nodding to the bed beside his, now empty. "That side of the room has a window. It would mean a lot to me. . . ."

"Of course," I say, berating myself for not having thought of this sooner. Of course, he should have a bed with a window. "I'll see to it right away."

I talk to the nurses, who are happy to oblige. A few hours later he's settled in the new bed, peering eagerly out the window. It's a lovely day outside, and he actually has a very nice view. He can see the light shining on the city, the nearby towers of a cathedral. I am momentarily amazed, as if he had managed to transport a piece of Valencia here, as if the sky were bluer out his window than anyone else's. I realize I can't remember the last time I saw the sun. Was that because of the long, gray Seattle winter, or have I just forgotten to look outside?

ONE AFTERNOON, I find a young man at his bedside, with a sensitive face and familiar sky blue eyes.

"This is my son," he says.

"I'd guessed." I introduce myself and reach out to clasp his hand.

"This is my doctor," Mr. Stone says seriously.

"Have you talked about—things?"

"Yes," says the father. "He knows. But you can tell him whatever you like."

"Do you . . ." I gesture broadly to the son. "Do you have questions about what's going on?"

"Not really," he says slowly. "I guess I understand."

I nod. "We can talk, if you find you have questions later on." I turn to his father. "Did the oncologists come in?" They were due this morning, to talk to him more about the diagnosis, the options for treatment, what he could expect.

"They were here earlier."

"Who?" the son asks.

"The oncologists. The cancer specialists," his father says.

"Do you want to talk about what they said to you?" I ask quietly.

"Not really."

I nod.

He sighs. "The same things we already knew. That given the size, and all the lymph nodes, there's not much they can do."

The son has fallen silent and looks ashen. He didn't know, I realize suddenly.

"I'm sorry," I say. "I thought—I thought you knew. Your father has metastatic lung cancer."

He nods very slowly, waits a long time before saying anything. "So . . . it's spread already?"

"Yes."

"Is surgery an option?"

I turn to the father. He's talked to the oncologists, I haven't yet. He shakes his head absently. "No. Chemo might buy a little time. We're going to talk about that further."

At this moment, of all moments, the shrill sound of a pager cuts into the silence, not my personal pager but the code pager.

"Code one ninety-nine, room three twenty-six C, CCU—"

I stare at it dumbly for a second, rooted to the ground. I look up at them.

"I—I have to go—" I get up, nod to both of them, and walk briskly out of the room. I keep myself from breaking into a run until the door is completely closed behind me.

I RETURN AS soon as the code is over.

"I'm sorry. There are a few things that happen in the hospital that you have to run to." I muster a smile.

"Is everything okay?"

"Yes." I'm lying. The man died, but there seems no point in saying this. "So—" I look up at the son, whose eyes are red and bright with tears. "Are you okay?"

He nods.

His father speaks the words I am about to say. "You didn't know?"

"No." I wonder what was said between them, that the son could not have heard what the father thought he'd said. I've learned over time that such misunderstandings are far from rare.

The father studies his son wonderingly. "You're very brave."

"Certain people throwing stones . . ." The son shakes his head.

"Bravery clearly runs in the family," I say. The same smile shines at me from two faces.

"I'm so sorry—If I had realized you didn't know, I would have tried harder to prepare you."

"This is the way I would have wanted to hear. With him."

"Still—I'm sorry," I say again.

WHEN I COME next, his son is gone.

"He seems like a lovely man," I say. "You must be proud."

He nods, but his expression turns serious. "I am. But I worry, too. He thinks he should take care of me, but I worry about him more than myself."

Sometimes, sitting at his bedside, I wonder who is really taking care of whom. I want to comfort him, to make all this easier, to keep him from being alone. Yet I sit beside him listening less out of courtesy or kindness than for my own pleasure. Even more than that—I want to learn from him. I am hungry for the knowledge he seems to have, of how to live a life you can be proud of at its end. After all, I am just embarking, full of uncertainty, into my own adult life, trying to forge the world in which I will live. I am trying to create my life, while he is looking back at his; and I would love to learn his lessons, to be able to feel when I am dying as fulfilled in what I have done as he is.

"I'm very lucky."

"So you keep saying." I smile at him.

"I—I wrote a book about the Basques. Not a long book. And not—not anything that most people would want to read. A scholarly work, you know."

I nod.

"It took me thirty-five years. The culmination of my life's work. But it was published, a few years ago. I did what I set out to do."

He nods quietly to himself, then a shadow crosses his face. "I won't see ninety," he murmurs, half to himself.

I look at him quizzically.

"I always thought I would live to be ninety—" He clears his throat. "Well," he says. "It wasn't important." He smiles at me sadly.

"But you have to make your teapot," I say.

"Indeed."

"Do you think you'll try to get back to Valencia?"

"I don't know," he says. "Right now—it would be impossible for me to go home. There would be no one to take care of me, like this. Right now it's just an impossible dream. But—we'll see."

He smiles, his bright, blinding smile.

HE'S WELL ENOUGH finally to go to the floor, where he'll stay for a few more days. Then he'll go home, until a decision is made about whether to try chemotherapy.

When it's time to move him downstairs, I make the calls to the person in charge of bed placement myself. "He's an old man," I say, although I don't really think of him that way. He's too vital for my idea of an old man. "He's dying of lung cancer. And it would make him so happy to have a room with a view—Something looking out over the harbor maybe; but anything with a window is okay. Please, it would mean so much—"

"We'll try," she says tiredly, not making any promises. They find him a single room, though, with a view of the water and the sunset.

HE SELDOM SEEMS sad. He seems to have no anger in him, and a remarkable amount of joy for someone who has just learned he is dying. His face seems to know no expression except a smile, though I catch him in a moment of sorrow now and then.

We are talking—he in his now accustomed loud whisper—about his friends in Valencia, about the dinners they would have, the wonderful food and wine, how they would sit in front of the fire and argue into the night about politics and history.

"I wish I would be able to talk again. . . ." His eyes are filled with an ineffable sadness, wistfulness, and I realize again how suddenly all this came upon him. He felt fine until a month ago, and now he'll never speak aloud again.

"I'm so sorry," I say, squeezing his hand, my eyes filling unexpectedly with tears.

"Bless you," he whispers.

HE SAYS "BLESS you" again, the day he goes home, as we are saying good-bye. I want to say, "You have blessed me, more than you know." But I'm afraid it will sound silly, so I try to put the thought in my eyes instead. I think he understands. He squeezes my hand one last time.

Other patients come, to fill his empty room, to fill my hours. But he stays with me, in the blue sky, in the lush greens and pinks of the spring that has finally come. I remember to look out the windows, to watch the evening light on the cathedral, which I still imagine as being magically transported from Valencia. And I hold his Spanish islands in my heart when there are moments I have trouble bearing, promising myself that I will go there someday, that I will walk along the cobbled paths and feel the sunshine and know the joy in my life that he had in his.

17. Out of Control

It is two minutes before 8:00 A.M. Morning rounds are about to begin, and we mill around the ICU, waiting for the team to converge. I am chatting with the fourth-year medical student, enjoying the rare quiet moment. Our team right now is very large and our patients very sick, and everything is starting to feel tinged with desperation, a sense of being out of control.

The pharmacist who is assigned to the team walks up, looking rather somber. We wish him a good morning.

"Mrs. Andrucelli died," he says solemnly in a low voice.

"Oh." We both frown. "I'm sorry—" I add.

"Last night," he says. "I guess it wasn't unexpected, but . . ."

He sighs and walks away. The medical student and I glance at each other surreptitiously.

There's a pause.

Then: "Who's Mrs. Andrucelli?" we each ask simultaneously.

"I don't know."

And then, on an impulse, which is no less irresistible for its inexplicability, we both start to giggle.

"What's so funny?" asks my resident, walking into the room.

I shake my head, try to stop laughing. "Hey, um, do you know Mrs. Andrucelli?" I break into giggles again, asking the question.

"Of course," she says. "I already heard—"

She looks at me strangely, as I try to contain my half-hysterical laughter. The medical student is giggling again also, and the resident stares from the one to the other of us, awaiting an explanation.

"She died on our service and . . . we don't even remember who she was. . . ." I choke out, still laughing.

The resident doesn't say anything, wisely choosing to wait for the hysteria to dissipate, then clears her throat for rounds to begin.

18. Complaints

Mr. Martin smoked two packs of cigarettes a day for forty years. He'd developed, needless to say, terrible emphysema. He was on a half dozen medications, but, as his primary doctor explained to me the day he was admitted, he periodically got tired of them. This was what happened a week or so before I met him. Predictably, his breathing deteriorated, until finally he came in, gasping for air. As we interviewed him in the ER, his breathing got rapidly worse and—despite multiple nebulizer treatments and intravenous antibiotics and steroids—he had to be intubated.

He spent a few days on the ventilator, slowly improving with steroids, antibiotics, frequent nebulizer treatments. On my day off, he was weaned off the vent. I walked in to his room in the ICU to preround the next morning. It's always a suspenseful moment, the first interaction with someone after he's been extubated; now that he can talk, you never know quite what he'll say, what he'll turn out to be like.

I look at him curiously, and he looks back, frowning.

"How are you doing?" I ask.

"Well, my throat hurts like hell— People have just been shoving tubes and shit down in there for some reason, and it *hurts,* and I'm probably going to have *scarring* back there and God only knows what, from you all shoving all these tubes around—"

He breaks off to glare at me.

"Mr. Martin, we put that tube down your throat because you weren't able to breathe and you were dying."

He snorts. He pauses for a second—just long enough to let me know that he's not even going to grace that comment with a response—then continues as if I hadn't said anything. "And I'm hungry, and I want to eat, and nobody will give me any food."

"How is your swallowing?" I ask. This is one of the items on my agenda.

"I swallow just fine if anyone would give me anything to swallow! But they just keep bringing me juice, and ice, and whatever."

They must have put him on a liquid diet, standard for someone who's just been extubated.

"So you haven't tried to swallow any solids yet at all?" I note this down.

"Well—" He pauses. I look up.

"Well . . . Yesterday I was so *hungry* and nobody would give me any food, so finally I just had my son go out and bring me in a hot dog. But no, you all haven't given me any solid foods yet, no."

I have to smile. I won't tell him this, but I'm hardly in a position to criticize. The closest I ever came to being hospitalized was as an undergraduate, when I spent a night in the student infirmary with a severe bout of the stomach flu. After being rehydrated, I quickly felt better and was ravenous. When they wouldn't feed me I had friends sneak in cookies and a candy bar, which went down fine. I felt much better afterward—not that I'm condoning such behavior. I was not in the ICU, I hadn't been near death the day before, and I hadn't just been extubated.

But still.

I change him to a regular diet, quickly before rounds so that he'll get a real breakfast.

ON ROUNDS WE discuss which antibiotic he should be on for his pneumonia. The pharmacist looks down at his patient information sheet and frowns. "You were talking about giving him a cephalosporin. You know he's penicillin allergic, and there's some cross-reactivity."

"He's not penicillin allergic," I say. "I remember asking that in the ER before he had to be intubated, and he gave a very definite no."

"Our records say he is," the pharmacist says.

"We'll ask again," says my resident.

We walk in, and he's eating breakfast. "Sorry to interrupt you. . . ."

He rolls his eyes.

"I've gone through with the team what we talked about earlier. I just have one quick question—"

"You have too many damn questions."

"Are you allergic to penicillin?"

"By God, can't you see I'm eating? You all just go away and come back sometime when I'm not eating, and then we can have a nice chitchat or whatever, but can you not see that I'm busy right now? Not that this food is anything to write home about, but I spent a long time waiting for it, and it ain't going to be any better cold."

Realizing that I'm fighting a losing battle, I leave him to finish his breakfast. Coming back after rounds and conferences, I walk into the room and discover that, by unfortunate coincidence, he's now in the middle of lunch.

"I can come back later."

"No, no, it's okay." He sighs tolerantly. "What is it?"

"Are you allergic to penicillin?"

"No."

"Are you sure?"

"Yeah, I'm sure. I mean, if you give me too much of it, it might be bad for me, but I'm not allergic to it, no."

Great.

"What happened when someone gave you too much of it?"

"Well, one time maybe someone gave me a whole lot of penicillin, and it didn't agree with my system, it was too strong for me, maybe. But if you gave me a regular amount it would be okay."

"What happened when they gave you too much?"

He rolls his eyes, pauses before answering. "I got this itchy rash all over. But hell, if you give me too much of anything something like that might happen, you understand?"

"Certainly," I say. "I understand."

I write "Penicillin allergy" on my note pad and underline it.

THE NEXT MORNING, for once, I go to see him after he's finished eating. The remains of his meal are sitting on the tray, well picked over.

"How was breakfast?" I ask, to open the conversation. I'm never sure what tone to strike with him. He's always griping—I haven't heard a neutral comment from him yet, much less a positive one. I'm pretty sure there's humor under his crabbiness, but I can never quite pin it down. I haven't managed to catch him in a laugh yet.

"Awful," he says. "You need a new cook. Whoever's down there doesn't know what the hell they're doing."

"I'll tell them that."

"You do that. I'll be waiting. You tell them I won't leave here until they start serving some decent food."

"I wouldn't hold my breath," I say.

IN A FEW DAYS, he's much better, doing well on oral steroids and antibiotics. I catch him, once again, in the middle of breakfast.

"How's your breathing?" I ask.

"Shitty. But no shittier than it always is."

"You feeling about ready to go home?"

"Hell yes. Anything to get away from you guys."

I listen to his lungs, check his vitals sheet, confirm that everything is going well. From his doorway, headed out, I turn back.

"Mr. Martin?"

"Yeah?"

"One more question."

"That's what you always say; 'just one. . . .' Do they teach you how to lie in med school? Okay, shoot."

"Has the food gotten any better?"

"*What?*"

"You said you weren't leaving till the food got better. Has it?" I maintain a deadpan, clinical expression.

He stares at me for a long moment. Finally he bursts out laughing. "How do you think I'll answer that. . . . Has the food gotten any better. You get out of here—"

I wave and walk away, listening to him laugh.

19. Death and the Oncologist

Yvonne Braun was dying. She had a widely metastatic adenocarcinoma, its site of origin unknown. She'd had a couple of rounds of chemotherapy with no response at all. She was admitted, the time I met her, because the tumor had invaded her spinal cord and paralyzed her legs. She came in for radiation therapy to her back—palliative treatment, hoping against hope to restore some temporary function to her legs. The treatment was unlikely to help, and didn't.

She was very young, only in her early fifties. In a dark twist of fate, her husband was also dying, a little more slowly than she, of lung cancer. They were devoted to each other. He spent as much time as he could at the hospital, and they were warm and loving together, beautiful to watch.

She was German by birth, and spoke with a lilting German accent. She had a calm, simple way about her that almost suggested naïveté. I was never sure how much of this was her true character, how much some side effect of the language barrier, or something else I didn't understand.

Every morning, as I finished prerounding, I would ask her if there was anything we could get for her. Every time she answered: "A new body?"

I would smile gently, and reply, "We'll order one up from Pharmacy," or some such thing.

Every morning on rounds my attending asked, "Do you have any questions?" and she said, "When will I be able to walk again?"

ONE DAY AFTER rounds, as I'm writing notes, Ellen, my attending, comes up behind me.

"You have Mrs. Braun's chart?"

I nod. She leans on the counter beside me, sighing heavily.

"I don't think she understands, really, what's going on here."

I'm not quite sure if she's talking to me or to herself. "No," I agree. "I know her primary oncologist has been talking to her, but . . ."

"They talked about code status, what to do if she has a sudden death," she agrees. "But I don't know if he talked to her, really, about what was going to happen."

"It's hard," I say. "It's so sad."

"It is hard. You don't want to take everything away from her. And yet we owe it to her to give her the truth, so she can decide what to do with the time she has."

She thinks for a minute, staring into space, her expression at once fierce and gentle.

"Come." She nods to me. I'm surprised. Attendings hardly ever invite me in for a discussion they're having with a patient, apart from rounds and family meetings. I set aside my charts to follow her.

Yvonne looks up, surprised, as we walk in. It isn't time for rounds or one of our usual visits. Ellen pulls a chair to her bedside, gestures me to get one also. "Is this an okay time to talk?"

Yvonne nods. Ellen pauses briefly.

"I just wanted to see—how you were feeling about things."

"Things?"

"Everything. All of this."

Yvonne waves her hand in a vague, helpless gesture. "I don't under-stand."

Ellen thinks for a moment, then speaks carefully. "As you know, you have a cancer that's going to kill you, sooner or later. I don't know if anyone's talked to you about that. I don't know how you feel, what you think about that, what questions you have."

Yvonne is silent for a long time before she speaks.

"I . . . I'm not ready," she says finally. "I'm afraid of dying—I don't know what it will be like. Well, I suppose no one does. . . ." A ghost of a smile drifts around her lips. "But I don't know how it happens. I mean, where does the cancer go?" She gestures vaguely to her chest, looks up at the doctor.

Ellen sighs. "There are different ways," she says slowly. "It's—it's not unlikely that you'll get an infection. That's most often how it hap-pens. Rarely it's something else—the tumor invades into an important blood vessel, or a part of the brain that makes you breathe. But infec-tions are more common."

Yvonne nods slowly. "I see."

There's a pause.

"So that's it," she says.

"What do you mean?" Ellen asks.

"Somehow I—I thought there would be more we could do." Her voice is distant, her eyes focused on something far away.

Ellen nods. "How does that make you feel?"

"Angry, I suppose," says Yvonne, a little absently.

"Angry—at the disease? Or the doctors? Or just angry generally?"

"Well—at the doctors, too, I guess. It just seems like you're giving up." Her word "you" hangs in the air. She does not meet Ellen's eyes, or mine.

"To have people be sick, and not to be able to do anything to help them—that's not why any of us went to medical school," says Ellen quietly. "We're angry, too. . . ."

"I got two rounds of chemo," Yvonne says. "There's a woman I met downstairs, she has breast cancer, and she got ten rounds. Why aren't you doing that with me?"

Ellen sighs. "The kind of cancer you have—it doesn't tend to respond well to chemotherapy."

" 'It doesn't tend to—' But how do you know, with me? Why don't you try?"

"We do know. Those two rounds that you got, that was us trying. And the cancer didn't respond at all."

Yvonne still looks unsatisfied.

"We could give you chemo," Ellen says gently. "We could keep giving it, even if it didn't do any good. But then what would happen is you'd get sick, and be in pain and throwing up and miserable, and even more likely to get an infection. And then you'd lose your chance to spend the time that you have at home, with the people you love, feeling as well as you can. Knowing that it wouldn't help, we don't want to take what you have away from you. That's why we're not doing chemo." Her voice is soft at the end, and full of pain.

Yvonne nods slowly, thoughtfully; and this time she seems to understand, to accept. "I see," she says.

Suddenly she smiles ruefully. "I suppose I'm hoping for a miracle. Some magic bullet." The smile fades a little, and she looks wistful.

"It's okay to wish for that. As long as it doesn't keep you from other things."

There's a long pause. "Well," Yvonne says resolutely, "why don't you let me just go home now? To take my few days and be there, at least. If there's nothing we can do."

"Oh." Ellen is suddenly almost brusque again. "I don't think it will be anything like that. I think you've got a lot more than a few days. Months, maybe."

Yvonne frowns doubtfully.

Ellen goes on. "I'm more worried about—I remember when you came in. We talked, and I asked you what you wanted. You told me what you wanted most of all was to get home. You talked about walking through the rooms of your house, about cooking with your husband. I remember how animated you were about that."

I catch myself being surprised, not having known they had a talk like that.

Yvonne nods sadly. "That was a long time ago."

"We are going to get you home—you understand that?" Her tone is fierce.

Yvonne looks uncertain.

"*You will go home.*" Ellen's voice brooks no uncertainty. "I'm just afraid that you won't be able to do what you'd been planning when you get there. Like walking. I don't think you'll be able to walk."

"Oh—" Yvonne thinks for a minute. "Well, that doesn't matter so much really. Just to make use of whatever I do have, and to be there, in my own place, and with my husband."

"You've got a wonderful husband. I was very much impressed by him."

Listening, I smile at her choice of words—*very much impressed.*

"I know," Yvonne says seriously.

"Good," Ellen says. "That's important."

"I wish we had more time together," she adds sadly.

"Many people never have any time with anyone who loves them that much," Ellen says quietly. "Lots of people never experience that at all. Remember that. You're lucky, too, as well as being unlucky. It's easy to get caught in 'why me?' But remember the other side of it, too."

Yvonne nods.

Ellen pauses. "Who else do you have, that's important to you?"

"Well, there's Mother . . ."

The obvious love in her voice is complicated by some other emotion—guilt? Fear? I can't exactly place the conflict that I hear, but Ellen's next question shows she does.

"Does she know how sick you are?"

"No. Not yet."

"When are you going to tell her?"

"It's not so simple. She's seventy-nine. She's still in Germany. I never envisioned it this way. I always thought it would be me going to her funeral, not the other way around—"

Her eyes fill with tears. "I don't want to hurt her. . . ."

I look up and see that there are matching tears in Ellen's eyes. She doesn't say anything, just reaches out to squeeze Yvonne's hand.

"I have a daughter," Yvonne adds quickly, as if unwilling to dwell on the subject of her mother.

"How old is she?"

"Thirty-one. She knows everything. She's been here a lot, helping. . . . She's a great strength to me."

Ellen pauses for a long moment. "Having a daughter—gives your life continuity."

Yvonne nods. "It's a wonderful thing to have a daughter. . . ."

I LOSE THE conversation for a second, swept back upon my own life and history. My mother had breast cancer, diagnosed when I was a first-year medical student. She's fine, but the special terror of the experience colors my interaction with cancer patients, especially women close to her age. It's impossible for me to see them and not imagine, fleetingly, her in their place. I find it harder to distance myself from their pain.

The connection here goes beyond cancer. My mother's mother died suddenly of a heart attack, in her early sixties. She and my mother had always had a tempestuous relationship; I know it is one of the enduring griefs of my mother's life that so much went unsaid between them on both sides. One of the most vivid pieces of family history I carry is the story of my grandmother at my mother's bedside when I was born. They had not known that I would be a girl, and when I emerged, my grandmother whispered: "You'll get to know what it's like to have a daughter." My mother says it was one of the only times she knew her mother was glad to have had her, glad to have a daughter.

On the other hand, she and I have learned the lessons of their difficult experience. If one of us were to drop dead tomorrow, there would be no doubt in either of our minds of how much we loved and were loved by the other, no words left unsaid.

Tangled in this web—Yvonne, her mother, and daughter; Ellen and whatever history guides her words; my own mother and grandmother—I have one of those moments of strange clarity when everything seems interconnected, tied into some deeper truth and meaning. I see an endless network of mothers, daughters, granddaughters, playing out the myriad dramas of that relationship. I see joy and regret, sickness and health, life and death, linked in their ever-turning cycles. We will each die in our time and our way, we each have our part to play on this stage. My head spins.

Can I imagine having to go to my mother's funeral? Worse yet—shifting generations, putting myself in Yvonne's place now—can I imagine what it would be like to know that my mother would have to go to mine?

ELLEN AND YVONNE continue to talk.

"This might be a time to say some of these things to your daughter," Ellen is saying.

"I already have."

"Good." Ellen nods, and reaches for her hand.

Looking up, Yvonne studies Ellen's face, her strong, gentle but serious expression, her eyes just a little red with drying tears. "How can you . . ." she asks suddenly. "I thought you weren't supposed to get emotionally invested in your patients." Her voice is tinged with wonder.

"You have to get emotionally invested," Ellen says. "It's the only way to be a doctor."

Yvonne nods.

We get up to go. I, the spectator, don't know what to say. I reach out and squeeze her hand. "We'll be here."

She squeezes back and nods.

IN THE HALLWAY Ellen turns to study me. I say nothing, but I see her taking in the raw emotion in my eyes.

"Are you okay?"

I nod. If I try to speak, I'll start crying.

"Here. Let's go to the lounge."

She takes me by the arm and I, soundless, let myself be guided to the patient lounge, a pleasant small half-enclosed space with a few sofas and a large window overlooking the water.

"Let me tell you a story."

I nod again.

"When I was an intern, on my oncology rotation, we had a patient—actually she was the other intern's patient, but she somehow gravitated more to me, I think because the other intern was a man, and she wanted a woman to talk to. Anyway, she attached herself more to me, and we talked a lot. She was very young—thirty-two—and she had breast cancer and she was dying. It was terribly, terribly sad. She had two young children, and she had been engaged to be married. And her fiancé, when he heard about the cancer—he just flipped out, he couldn't deal with it. He disappeared."

I take a deep breath.

"So it was awful."

I nod, and she continues.

"It was Christmastime. And on Christmas, I go into her room, and she has this diamond necklace, in the shape of a snowflake—it's gorgeous. She pulls it out from around her neck to show to me; 'Look what I have.'

"And I say, 'It's beautiful; where did it come from?' And she says, 'My fiancé gave it to me.' So—you know he's back."

I smile, brushing away the tears that keep fighting toward my eyes, and she pauses a long moment.

"And then she says: 'Do you think I'll be well enough in March to have the wedding?'

"March was when they had been supposed to get married. Before all this happened." She takes a deep breath. "It's December. You have no idea how terminal she was—I mean, really. Just slipping away.

"What do you say? I have no idea what I even said. Whatever I could think of to get through the moment somehow. And I went back to the residents' room, and I just lost it. The rest of the team came in and I was there, sobbing, and they were like, what, what? And I told them, and you know what they said? They said: 'If you're that thin-skinned, if you're going to let things get to you like that, you shouldn't be in medicine.'

"That's what they said. And I spun on them and I said: 'If I ever stop letting things get to me, that's when I'll quit medicine.'

"And it turned out the chief resident of psychiatry was sitting there, listening to all this—I hadn't even seen him—and he stood and said, 'That's the sanest thing I've heard all week.'"

I smile through the tears that are rolling down my cheeks again.

"It's not a bad thing to cry, okay? More than that: it's the right thing. It's what you need to do—for yourself, and for your patients, too. Don't give that up, okay? Don't let anybody talk you out of it."

I nod.

"Sit here for a bit, if you need to, all right?"

I nod again. "Thank you . . ." The words come out scratchy and faint.

She nods and walks away.

I sit on the sofa silently for a minute. Then I reach for the telephone, to call my mother and tell her that I love her—even though I know she already knows.

20. Good-byes

A week later Ellen goes back to her lab, replaced by a more distant attending. I am on my own again, trying to find some way to keep my heart and mind functioning even though each feels stressed to breaking.

"What do you know about dying?" Yvonne asks me one day, out of the blue. I've come by at the end of the day before going home, to say hello, see if she needs anything.

I take in a sharp breath, then let it out again. "I've seen some people go through it," I say slowly.

"Tell me about it."

"What do you want to know?" I ask.

She shrugs. "What happens?"

Don't ask me this, I want to plead. *Don't ask me these things*

Instead I say, "Usually it's very quiet. We're very good at controlling pain, at the end. . . ."

Her eyes are wide as she stares at me. "Tell me more," she says.

"What do you want to know?"

"What do people actually die of?"

I sigh. "Different things. Often it's an infection, a pneumonia or something else, that gets out of control. Or the tumor itself can invade into a critical place, like the center in the brain that controls breathing."

She continues staring at me, unspoken questions burning through her eyes.

"All of those things are usually very peaceful. If someone has pain or trouble breathing, we have medications to control those. Usually at the end, the blood pressure just drops too low, and then people stop breathing and their hearts stop, and it's very quiet."

I've seen other kinds of death—the fire-and-brimstone kind, people throwing up blood and drowning in it, all kinds of horrible things. But I don't tell her this.

She nods slowly, and is quiet for a long time.

"I'm not ready to die," she says softly.

"I know."

"My mother is back in Germany. I—I haven't told her. She doesn't know. She's an old woman, she doesn't have the energy or the strength to come."

I reach out and take her hand.

"I was supposed to go to her funeral. I was supposed to help her die. Children are supposed to have to deal with their parents dying. Not the other way around."

I have identified her with my mother from the beginning, but now I connect her with myself. What would it be like for my mother to watch me die? Or to be six thousand miles from my nearest flesh and blood, rushing toward death, and not even have her know.

"And my daughter. I was supposed to help her raise my grandchildren! I had so many things to tell her, to tell them. So many things I wanted to do with them while they were growing up. And now it's all gone, all lost."

There is nothing I can possibly say, so I just sit there on the side of the bed, holding her hand, feeling the tears rush to my eyes and letting them fall.

She looks up at me, and an expression like wonder crosses her face, a strange tenderness. "Do you—cry a lot of tears?"

I'm not sure how to answer this. "There are so many things in life that deserve tears," I say.

A FEW DAYS later I'm on call, and I'm having a terrible day. My pager seems to go off every few seconds. A patient pulls out an NG tube that we had just spent two hours putting in. Someone else tears her special chemo line, which no one including me knows how to handle, necessitating a dozen phone calls before we can sort out what to do. Meanwhile, there are all the usual things: transfusions to order, electrolytes to replace, fevers to evaluate. None of these are crises, but a thousand small things need attention. "Mr. Johnson needs his lotions for his feet, but he doesn't know what they're called." Or, "The guy in six sixty-nine lost his IV and we can't get another one in and he's throwing up."

In the midst of all this, a nurse grabs me in the hall. "Mrs. Braun says she has to see you, right away."

I take a breath that is part sigh, part groan. "I can't go right now. Tell her I'll be there as soon as I can."

"Okay."

As I turn to walk away, the nurse clears her throat. "Umm . . ." She seems uncertain whether to go on. "She said—she said she wants to ask you how she can die with dignity."

I look up. "What?"

"Well—that's what she said. She won't eat, and she's not sure she wants the electrolytes and the fluids that were ordered. I thought you should be prepared."

I back against the wall and close my eyes for a second. Part of me wants to cry and part to laugh. Here I am with a thousand detailed questions swirling in my mind and now, at this particular moment on this particular night, Mrs. Braun needs to know how to die with dignity. Can I just write for that in the order book? "Death with dignity, please."

"Tell her I'll be there in a little bit," I repeat, opening my eyes. I add, wearily, "And . . . thanks for the heads-up."

As soon as I can, I go in to her room.

"I. . . . I need to talk," she says.

"Yes," I say, trying not to sound fatigued.

She hangs her head. "The nurse said you were very busy."

I shake my head. "It's okay," I say.

"I'm sorry I'm making things so hard for everybody," she says.

"You don't need to be sorry for anything. You're not, and even if you were, you shouldn't apologize."

"The nurse came with all those medicines. She said my potassium and magnesium are off again, and I'll need a blood transfusion soon."

I nod.

She sighs. "I just—I don't know if I should be doing all these things. What's the point? I'm just going to die anyway, so what's the point in bothering? Shouldn't I just—get it over with?"

There are moments when I am struck dumb by the things that people say to me, the questions that they ask.

"Yvonne, dear—it's up to you, you know that. I can't tell you how much time you have. The point of the medicines is that you thought you wanted most to get home and that can't happen without them. That doesn't mean you have to take them, but it's the reason you should think about it."

"Going home . . . I was beginning to think maybe that was just a silly dream. That it could never really happen." Her voice is dreamy, distant.

"It's not a dream," I say, perhaps more forcibly than I ought. "It's a plan. It's always impossible to make promises, but if that is what you want, I am going to do everything in my power to make it happen. And I think it will."

I listen to myself with a certain alarm. Have I internalized this too much, have I made getting her home my own goal rather than hers? She was so animated when she talked about it. And what I see in her eyes now is not resignation but despair.

"What should I do?" she whispers.

"Only you can answer that. But I think you should try not to give up."

She thinks for a while. "I think . . . I think I'll eat my dinner."

"I think that's a great idea."

"I wasn't going to. But I will."

She looks up suddenly as I'm leaving. "How old are you?"

I've learned that this isn't a question I have to answer. "Old enough not to tell people how old I am." I smile at her affectionately.

"But I'm old enough to be your mother!" she protests.

You're the same age as my mother. It occurs to me, for the hundredth time, to say to her: *My mother has had cancer, too.* Fast behind this impulse always comes another one, advising me to keep this piece of information to myself. The doctor-patient relationship is mutual but not symmetric. I can bring my emotions and personal life to it in limited ways, in ways that can help me to help her, but some fears are too raw for me to lay on the table. I can't risk putting her in the position of feeling she needs to help or comfort me.

A little while later her nurse stops me again, in the rush of managing details. "What did you say to Mrs. Braun?"

I suddenly can't think of an answer. "I told her if she'd let us get her through this, I thought she could go home to spend some time and then die there, and that would be best."

"Oh." She looks largely, but not completely, satisfied.

"She told me you told her to eat," she says.

"Something like that." I smile.

I go in later, when my night has calmed down a little, to make sure Yvonne is still all right.

"I had a good conversation with my daughter tonight," she says, her smile tired but genuine.

"Good," I say.

"We talked about all kinds of things. There's so much I feel I have to say. While I still can."

I nod.

"It's just all so hard," she says.

"I know," I say.

"Oh, just tell me what to do—" she says, desperation tinging her voice again, her eyes filling with tears.

I sigh. I'm sitting at the edge of her bed, and I reach out to brush the hair out of her eyes. "Sleep," I say. "That's all the advice I have for tonight. Just sleep."

Slowly she nods, then closes her eyes. I watch her until her breathing becomes slow and steady, then slip out of the room.

It's late spring. The days are long in Seattle at this time of year, and the sun has not yet set. Furtively, I slip out the back door of the hospital. This entrance opens onto a narrow park along the wall of the ship canal. You can walk there, navigating among the geese and their goslings, ducking under the willow boughs that hang over the edge of the water. Boats go by, under sail or motor or oar. The water is deep by the reinforced bank, and some boats come so close you could almost jump onto them. I fantasize about this sometimes, what would happen if I hopped onto a passing vessel, white coat and scrubs and all, sailed away onto the clear blue sea, tossing my pager into the wake behind me.

Farther along, the path passes under a drawbridge. You can stand below it as it opens, watch the huge, graceful lattice lift and stretch into the air. I study the mechanism, note the heavy counterweights and the way that the two halves connect and disconnect. I am awed by the loveliness of the structure, and I remember how I once thought of becoming an engineer. How different my life would be if I had chosen that path instead of this one.

On the far side of the bridge, you step out into sunlight, a bright round bay lined with tall grasses. The beauty of the mountains on the other side of the lake notwithstanding, I am only a ten-minute walk to a telephone, if my pager goes off.

I will always love this hospital for this: the park and the water, the flowers, the willow. The gentle reminder contained in the bridges, the boats, the houseboats: that life goes on, on the outside, that for all the tragedies we see, there are simple, healthy dramas playing out in the world beyond the hospital walls. There's joy, health, normalcy out there. So often, where I live and work, it's hard to believe that. This little walk in fresh air scented with flowers restores my faith more than almost anything. I contemplate the strange truth that the sun will shine after Yvonne is gone.

WHEN IT BECOMES clear that the radiation is not going to restore function to Yvonne's legs, we begin making arrangements for her to go home. We set up visiting nurses and home health workers to assist her, and order a special bed which she can get in and out of easily. The physical and occupational therapists work intensively with her and her husband to help prepare them for the needs of daily life. She'll have ongoing therapy at home, as well.

And then, on the morning she's supposed to leave, all hell breaks loose.

It happens during morning rounds. My team and I are in a room two doors down from hers with another patient. A nurse slips in and tugs my sleeve.

"It's Mrs. Braun—"

"We should be there in just a minute."

"You need to come now."

I race with her to Yvonne's room, where a few nurses are already hovering. Yvonne is slumped over a little on the bed, looking greenish, her skin damp and pasty. I ask how she's feeling, and she can barely spit out the word: "Sick . . ." The nurse informs me that her blood pressure is seventy over palp, barely measurable.

"Oxygen," I say. "Get a monitor. Start an IV, we need fluids—"

She looks terrible. She's completely limp now and her eyes are closed. "Yvonne," I say. "Yvonne, hold on."

It feels like minutes pass, though it's only a few seconds. Someone is telling me that they're looking for a monitor but can't find one, and a young nurse is poking Yvonne's arm over and over with an IV but can't get it in. And she's dying in front of my eyes, and I don't know what to do.

Where the hell is my team? I stick my head out into the hallway—they've got to be out there talking, where else could they be? But there's nobody. Then the social worker walks by and says rounds were running late, so the team headed off to radiology conference. I'm supposed to meet them there, she says. We'll finish rounding later.

"Fuck," I whisper.

I tell a nurse to page my resident and tell him that I need him, now.

The monitor has finally arrived and shows sinus tachycardia, a very rapid heart rate. I'm yelling again for fluids, which still aren't running. My mind is racing along a different course, however. I wonder what I have done wrong to bring her here, what I could have done to foresee or prevent this. I was in charge of her, so surely this was somehow my fault.

And, if possible, even a worse thought: I promised her she could go home. I promised her time, even if it was only a little time. I'd offered such a small thing in exchange for the whole life she was giving up. What was I going to do if I couldn't deliver?

My resident walks in, sharp and efficient as always.

"What's going on?" he asks.

"Her—her blood pressure's down. She was sitting up and suddenly she said she felt sick and keeled over. She's—we're—I've started oxygen and fluids, she's in sinus tach—"

"What's your differential diagnosis?"

I sputter. "God, um, infection, sepsis, some neuro thing from her tumor, an MI or a pulmonary embolus I suppose—"

"What antibiotics do you want to start empirically at this point?"

I stare at him.

"What organisms are you trying to cover?"

What organisms, what organisms, what organisms . . . The words spin and swim in my head. What organisms—

My resident shakes his head impatiently. "What do her labs show?"

"We're still getting them," I say. "The nurse is having trouble accessing her vein—"

"If you can't get a peripheral stick, you need to go for the femoral."

I nod dumbly. I've always hated getting blood from the femoral vein, a big vein in the groin. It's supposed to be easy. I can hit a hard vein like the subclavian on the first try, no problem, but I've never been consistent with the femoral.

She doesn't have enough pressure to have a pulse to guide me. So I am stabbing at her groin, blindly, and no blood comes. And worse—much worse—she is not moving, not flinching, not reacting at all as my needle moves in and out of her flesh.

My resident stares at me and suddenly says perhaps the worst thing that anyone has ever said to me. "Where did you go to medical school?"

And I don't say, I went to Dartmouth. And I aced both Medicine and Surgery. And they used to call me in the middle of the night when the IV nurses couldn't get a stick, because I could get blood out of a stone. So fuck off.

I don't say anything. I just keep poking desperately in Yvonne's groin. And suddenly there's blood in the tube. And just as suddenly, the crises passes. She opens her eyes, and her blood pressure rises, and she still looks shaky and pale, but the terrible moment has passed.

My resident shrugs and heads back to rounds. I stay with Yvonne. She's still trembling, and we're still waiting for a chest X-ray and labs and an EKG.

"I want to talk to my husband," she says.

"I don't think this is the best time for that," I say. "Okay? You can call him in just a little bit, when everything is settled."

"I need to talk to him now." Her voice breaks pathetically on the last word.

"What do you need to say?" I ask gently.

"I just need to tell him what's going on." She meets and holds my eye.

Against my better judgment, I lift the phone. She tells me the number, and I dial for her before handing her the receiver.

"Darling?" She gulps. "It's me."

There's a pause.

"I'm not going to make it," she says in a tiny voice. "I just called to say good-bye. . . ."

Jesus fucking Christ! I spin on her.

"Tell him you had a reaction," I say in a steely voice, resisting the impulse to yell.

"The doctor says I had a reaction," she says faintly.

"Tell him it's going to be okay."

"She says it's going to be okay."

"Give me the phone."

She holds it up innocently, and I grab it. He's sobbing, of course, on the other end.

"Please—" I say.

"What's happening?" he almost screams.

"I'm so sorry," I say. "I didn't realize she was going to say that, or I would have talked to you myself. She's having a little trouble. She was feeling sick and her blood pressure was low. But she's doing a lot better, and we're giving her fluids and antibiotics, and we're doing tests to find out exactly what happened. We'll know more in a little while. But she's a lot better, and it's very important not to panic."

"I'm sitting here waiting for the bed—" His voice breaks on every other word. "The fucking hospital bed that she was supposed to have when she comes home. I'm sitting around waiting for the goddamn delivery people and she's in there dying—"

"She isn't dying," I repeat. "I don't think she's in a critical situation right now. She won't be able to come home today, but we really can't tell anything more than that yet—"

"Then I don't need the damn bed. . . ."

"Why don't you come in," I suggest. "We'll know more very soon. But please, try not to panic. We just need to take care of her right now. But she's going to be okay."

As SUDDENLY AS she got sick, she came back to normal. The episode passed completely within half an hour. We never found out exactly what had happened; her cultures were all negative for infection, her cardiac studies were normal. It could have been an infection that we never found. It might have just been something similar to a faint, a momentary instability in the nerves that help maintain blood pressure. Whatever it was, it didn't happen again.

The next afternoon everything is completely back to normal, we're working again to get things ready for her to go home. I walk into the room and find her husband at her bedside. I apologize profusely for the terrible telephone conversation. We find ourselves recapping the events of the day before.

"If I had known what you were going to say, I never would have given you the phone." I smile at her scoldingly. I'm amazed that we can talk about this now, this way, so soon.

"Well—you said it wasn't critical. To me it was critical." Her voice holds just the faintest hint of accusation.

I sigh. "I know. I don't at all mean to be denying that. It's just I didn't want him to think you were dying, when you weren't."

"That's exactly what I thought," he says, his voice breaking on the words. I remember the ache in his voice the day before.

"I thought I was," she says softly.

"I know."

She smiles at me as she releases my hand. Then she turns to her husband. "That other doctor was trying to make her decide what to do. He kept yelling questions at her, and frowning. He was mean."

"Maybe he just didn't know what to do," her husband suggests. "Maybe he didn't have the authority."

"No," I break in. "It's the other way around. He was trying to get me to work through it. He was reminding me that I won't always have someone there to help me, as I do now. He was doing it to teach me. It's okay. It's a good thing."

Yvonne wrinkles her nose dubiously, and I have to smile. Underneath, I'm reeling with the impact of what she's just revealed. While I had thought she was too sick to be aware of much, in fact she had watched the whole incident, me stunned and stumbling, not knowing what to do. I remember her lying still and uncomplaining through my attempts at a femoral stick, and I realize that she wasn't too dazed to care. She was protecting me.

Even more amazing: she doesn't judge me for it. The comfortable, competent management of a crisis is not, to her or to her husband, essentially what it means to be a doctor, to be *her* doctor. This thing that seems so central, so critical, to me, isn't what they care about. My doctorhood is something completely different to them, though at this moment I don't understand what it possibly could be.

"I'll see you before you go, to say good-bye," I promise. She nods. I'm not sure what I'm going to say.

When I walk into her room a few hours later, the bed is empty, stripped. A nurse glances in. "The ambulance came early," she says. "Her husband was here, and she was ready. So she went."

I nod.

"I'm sorry," she says hesitantly, catching the look in my eye.

"It's okay."

21. Homage

I will begin with a confession: I used to find the two men comical. They were so very old, so perfectly matched in their white-haired, white-coated paleness, such an epitome of the medicine of generations ago. They reminded me of the old pair in black suits on the Muppets, or a couple of twinned Mr. Burnses from the Simpsons, whom they did physically resemble. They came to noon conference, the daily lunch-and-lecture otherwise attended exclusively by the residents, the pack of us in our youth and cockiness and book-learning that outweighed our clinical expertise. They came religiously, day after day, sat near the front of the small room and listened earnestly, and frequently asked questions: strange questions, often, antiquated to the rest of us, sometimes almost foolish to those with a more current medical school education, sometimes unexpectedly adroit.

I sometimes wondered, affectionately yet with a certain condescension, whether they thought that this was sufficient; that coming to conference for an hour five times a week could keep them current in the cutting edge of medicine. I admired their coming but wondered what they got from being there.

Over time, the amusement diminished and the admiration grew. The old men were different from anyone I'd ever known. They were tentative, lacking the unflappable serenity of the old country docs I knew in med school. They didn't seem quite at peace with medicine and their role in it, willing to accept that their glory time had passed and was fading now, but still struggling with the need to understand, to know more, to delve deeper. They knew that things had changed, but weren't willing just to be left behind.

I learned to listen more closely to their questions. They were strange, yes, but they had kernels of truth to them, displaying a wonderful clarity of thought. I started to realize that the very magnitude of the difference between their perspective and mine increased what I could learn from them. There were things that were clear in their sight that were confused in mine, as much as the other way around. I learned to be glad when their pale, polite hands went up, to know that something interesting would follow.

I didn't discover any more about them—their names, their histories—until one fateful day late in my internship year. I had just come back to the university hospital, to be on the Hematology/Oncology, or "Heme/Onc," service. I'd only been there a few days, and had barely had time to note the absence of the old men from noon conference.

One of the other interns was telling me about his patients before he went home for the night.

"Then there's Dr. Williams," he said, dropping his voice.

"Yes?" I said.

"You've heard he has metastatic prostate cancer?"

I frowned, uncertain. "I'm sorry—is he someone I should know?"

"Dr. Williams. You know, Dr. Williams."

"I do?"

"The old guy. You know the old guys from lunch conference."

My heart sank suddenly. *"Oh."*

"You don't know who he is? He used to be one of the top deans of the med school. He was quite the muckety-muck. And you know Dr. Paulson?"

I frowned again, not recognizing the name.

"The other one. The one he was always with at conference."

"Sure."

"He's the guy who invented the Paulson-Ames test." He named a lab test we all use every day.

"You're kidding."

"I'm serious."

"You've got to be kidding."

"Nope."

"Wow. I had no idea."

"Giants. Those guys are giants." He paused. "Anyway—Dr. Williams has prostate cancer. He had surgery and radiation, but recurred. It's been progressing fast over the last few months—he's not doing very well."

DR. WILLIAMS struggled on for several weeks, his condition slowly worsening. One night, his intern said, before he left, "I think he might die tonight."

I nodded.

"There may be issues that will come up for you," he went on. "He's too sick to really communicate anymore. He's breathing really fast, and I think he's uncomfortable. But the family's been concerned about giving him too much medicine and hastening things. So—I don't know. Just play it by ear. The family has been here a lot, just try to work with them. . . ."

IT WASN'T LONG before I got the call. The nurse said Dr. Williams had a respiratory rate in the forties, about twice normal, and looked quite uncomfortable. The family was with him and wanted to talk.

His wife and two sons were there, although one son did most of the talking. I was tentative, partly because of the other intern's warning, partly because I always am when talking to families whose loved ones are dying. I think it's because in this, more than in almost anything else, I want to be sure not to impose my will on theirs. Trying to uncover their thoughts, to discover their leanings and then officially concur with their chosen path, is a delicate business. You float ideas and gauge reactions, always ready to pull a half-suggestion back if it seems not to suit. There are certain careful, guarded phrases which mark these discussions, lots of "probables" and "possibles" and "I think" and "I really doubt." No definites for the dying.

They asked me whether I thought we should start a morphine drip. I chose my words carefully. "I think—that he's not very aware of what's going on right now. So in a certain sense, it probably doesn't make a great deal of difference which path we choose. I think it won't be very much longer either way. I don't think he's alert enough to suffer."

They nodded, both absorbing and seeming to agree. I tried to read their faces, to guess what they wanted, which way I should be helping to lead them. They seemed to be waiting for me to say something more.

"On the other hand, it's possible that his rapid breathing and fast heart rate are on some level an indicator of discomfort. If we were to give him something to slow those down, it might be easier for him."

His son nodded thoughtfully.

"Would you like us to go ahead and do that?"

The three of them looked at each other. Slowly they nodded.

"Okay," I said gently. I took a deep breath, looked up, glanced at each of them. "We—we all know him, all admire him. It's hard for us to see him this way. I can only imagine how it must be for you. We all are grieving with you."

Not sure what if anything more to say, I turned and walk out.

I wrote for a morphine drip at a low dose. His breathing slowed to a more normal rate, and he looked considerably more comfortable. I studied the family with equal attention. They seemed more comfortable, too. I took a slow sigh of relief.

It was only an hour or so later that the nurse called back. "Dr. Williams's son came out to say his father passed."

I worried that they might be upset, might think the morphine had hurried the process. Though tearful, they seemed okay. The three of them were in the room, stroking his hands and his forehead, their expressions at once sad and peaceful.

"Are we allowed to stay with him for a little bit?" they asked.

"Of course," I said.

"Thank you—"

I busied myself with paperwork to let them be alone. A while later, I thought I saw them walking down the hallway, so I slipped in to do the quick exam that documents a death. The son was still there by his father's bedside.

"I'm sorry—" I started to back out. "Take all the time you need."

"No, it's okay. What do you have to do?"

"Just a very brief exam."

"Go ahead," he said gently.

I stepped to the bedside, performed the now-familiar ritual of checking heart, lungs, reflexes. I stepped back.

He cleared his throat. "Could we—you know. Get rid of some of this." He nodded to the oxygen tubing around his father's nose and chin, the IV pole and pump.

"Of course."

Feeling strangely awkward, I fumbled. The oxygen was easy, but when I unhooked the IV it started dripping, and I couldn't figure out how to turn it off. Finally I gave up and dragged the pole and pump clumsily into the hall. I groaned silently at myself. I am not at my most graceful at three-thirty in the morning. But it was done, and I left the son alone with his father's body.

On the day after Dr. Williams died, I saw Dr. Paulson, at lunchtime, walking not into conference but into the cafeteria. He was beside someone, but seemed to my prejudiced eye suddenly and terribly alone. It occurred to me that this was the first time I'd seen him without Dr. Williams at his side. A shudder of grief passed through me, and I wanted to reach out and touch him, say that I had been there at the death, that I was sorry. That we were all sorry for his loss, for his new and awful loneliness, that we hoped he would keep coming to our conference.

Uncertainty and the awkwardness of the moment stopped me, and he passed on into the cafeteria, while I went on to the lecture alone.

I thought for a few days that I would regret that moment forever. But a week or so later I was standing in the lunch line at the conference when a familiar form appeared beside me. "Hi," I said, smiling. I'd never talked to him before.

"Looks good," he said, surveying the pasta and salad.

"It does," I agreed.

We sat down together, to listen to the presentation.

22. The Last Night

I was on call on the last night of internship. I had been counting down the hours for a week. Now it was 8:00 P.M., and in twelve hours I would hand off the pager to a wide-eyed new intern. Another July.

But tonight there was a man dying down the hall. He had lung cancer, widely metastatic. Until a few hours ago it wasn't clear whether he had days left or months. Earlier in the day he was walking, talking, smoking cigarettes. But then his temperature spiked high and his breathing slowed and he slipped into a coma.

I called his brother.

"It's time to come?" he said.

"Yes."

Now I was lying on the bed in my call room, waiting. Hoping that the next page would be for the brother's arrival, not for the patient's death.

My friend Chris from the gym had the final two days of internship off. He paged me, drunk and sentimental, with loud party noises in the background.

"Em, we made it. I just can't believe we made it."

"We made it," I echoed, looking around me at the call room. *I haven't quite made it yet*, I thought.

"And now it's over, and we never have to do it again. Sure, there's the rest of residency, but we never have to be interns again."

My pager went off.

"I could never have done it without you," he said.

"And I couldn't have without you. We did it together."

"I just can't believe it's over."

My pager beeped again.

"I have to go, okay?"

"I wish you were here celebrating," he said.

"Me too."

The loudspeaker crackled on. "Code one ninety-nine, room three fifty-three C."

"I really have to go now, okay?"

"Okay. Have a good night."

"Have a good one for me."

I put down the phone and ran.

The code wasn't for my patient—he didn't want anything done, when the time came. It was for a patient on the cardiology service, and it went well: we got a pulse back. The cardiologist swept him off to the catheterization lab to try to open his blocked heart vessel.

I went back to my call room and sat on the cot with the lights out. The window showed an ink blue sky, the profile of trees, a single star. I closed my eyes, savoring the quiet of the call room, the calm before the

126

storm. Never before this year had I so appreciated silence, or the value of a small and temporary refuge.

Next year would be different. There would be interns to take care of. I would become a supervisor, with the good and bad changes that implied. I would have less detail work, fewer pages in the night for little things; those would go to the interns. I would get to do more teaching. But by moving up on the totem pole I would lose my place at the front line of patient contact: the interns would do the initial interviews, the daily checkups, while I listened and supervised. I would miss that intimacy with my patients, though I wouldn't miss the 3:00 A.M. calls for Tylenol and sleeping pills.

The pager went off. My patient's brother had arrived. I turned the light back on and adjusted my wrinkled scrubs.

Eight more hours.

23. Sudden Death

He comes in at one in the morning, after calling the medics for chest pain and dizziness. They found him at home in new-onset atrial fibrillation, with a very fast heart rate and a blood pressure too low to measure. They gave him fluid and oxygen. By the time he gets to us, he's doing better.

He's a small, quiet man, with gentle but reserved eyes, who responds with few words to my many questions.

"I'm cold," is the only thing he offers on his own, murmured softly toward the end of the interview.

"I just need to have a quick look and listen to you," I say. "Then we'll get you upstairs where it's warmer."

As I pull back the sheet, I am shaken by his thinness, ribs delicately carved in skin, the triangular xiphoid bone at the base of his rib cage a prominent arrow. His belly is terribly sunken though not tender, his hipbones protrude in a graceful but disturbing arc.

"Have you lost weight recently?" I ask.

"I don't weigh myself," he answers diffidently.

"I understand," I say. "But do you have a sense of it? Do your clothes fit differently? Have you changed belts or the notch you use?"

"Everything's about the same," he says. "I've always been skinny." He looks down placidly at his emaciated body.

"How's your appetite?"

"I eat okay," he says. "Not much of a cook, but I eat."

Nothing else of interest shows up in his history or physical. I give him medications to control his heart rate, and he converts back into a sinus rhythm overnight. I make sure that he hasn't had a small heart attack, check a wide array of lab tests—blood counts, thyroid tests—all of which are normal. He stays in sinus rhythm.

I call his outpatient attending. "He came in for a-fib, and that seems to be resolved now. He converted spontaneously, and our workup for secondary causes has been negative."

"Good," he says.

I'm not quite sure what to say next. "I just wanted to touch base with you. . . . He's awfully thin. He just doesn't look healthy." My words sound painfully unprofessional to me—couldn't I come up with something more technical?—but that's the truth, he just looks bad.

"I know," he says. "He's always been like that, as long as I've known him, anyway. I did a chest X-ray—you probably repeated it—and basic labs, which were all fine. I think he's just skinny. Ask him, he says he's always been skinny. . . ."

"Always been skinny," I repeat, half to myself. Is anyone always that skinny? I suppose so. . . .

" Let me know when he's leaving, I'll make sure to get him in soon," he says.

LATER, A NURSE ON his floor pulls me aside. "What does the little guy in room eight have?"

"A-fib," I say. "He's out of it now."

"He doesn't eat much of anything."

"I know."

"He looks like he came out of a concentration camp."

It's hard to dispute this. "I understand that you're worried. So am I."

"You heard about his wife?" she says.

"No," I say, startled.

"Oh, I was just talking to him. His wife has Alzheimer's, pretty bad it sounds like. He does everything for her: washes her, dresses her, feeds her. Pretty amazing for a guy who looks on his last legs, himself."

"That's so sad."

"I asked if anyone comes in to help, and he said no," she continues. "I told him we could arrange that, and he just shook his head and wouldn't talk about it anymore. He's proud, I think, under that sweet exterior. Who knows what he's going through."

I TRY ASKING about his life at home, about his wife; but he says they're doing fine and that he doesn't want to talk about it. The finality in his tone, the frown that accompanies his words tell me not to push; and I don't, although I wonder how much he's holding inside, and whether there's any way to reach or to help him. I run through screening questions for depression, but the answers all suggest he doesn't have it. He's coping well with whatever he has to deal with.

We keep him for a couple of days, trying to get him to eat more, waiting for him to seem stronger, more well. I know I should send him home—we aren't doing much but pushing food on him—but something in me demurs. Something feels wrong. I tell myself that his outpatient doc will keep following him, that I don't have to solve every problem while he's in the hospital, that I need to learn to let go.

ON THE MORNING he's supposed to go home, I come in to find my sign-out sheet lying on my desk. There on the page are the notes I wrote about him for the person covering overnight; a list of his problems and medications, and "Nothing to do, waiting to go home" penned in the box of the night's plans. Under it in the covering resident's neat script is written: "Deceased. See note."

I freeze, staring uncomprehendingly at the three words. I stop breathing, my vision blurs. "Deceased."

It is hard to explain how, even in the hospital where death is hardly a rarity, a sudden death can still be so completely shocking. Perhaps in fact it is especially shocking here—at home, unwatched, it's somehow more acceptable for people to suddenly drop dead. But here? I'm supposed to know everything about my patients, I'm supposed to have it all in hand. People may still die, but if they do it should be from things I know and understand, battles we have fought and declared lost. By some unspoken but absolute code, patients are allowed to die in the hospital, but only if it's planned.

I can't count the number of patients I've had die so far in residency, but this is the first one to die without my predicting it. Moreover, I'm at the beginning of my second year now; I'm no longer an intern, I no longer have a senior resident looking over me. I'm newly in charge, a frightening enough thing in itself—and now this happens.

I FIND THE patient's chart, read the brief note from the covering resident; it describes the code and documents the death, not much else. My heart in my throat, I find the resident and ask what happened.

"He just—coded," he says. "The nurse went in and found him not breathing." He sighs. "I'm not sure how long he'd been dead. He wasn't on a monitor anymore, and they hadn't checked on him in an hour or so. Anyway, we coded him for a while, but never got a rhythm back."

"I'm sorry," I murmur.

"No, I'm sorry," he says. "I wish we could've got him back."

"It's okay," I say. "It's not your fault."

"HE JUST CODED." My voluble imagination races with this. What could have killed him out of the blue like that? What could I have missed, or worse yet, what could I have done?

A pulmonary embolus, always first on the differential of sudden death, a clot that went to his lungs—was I giving him something to prevent that? I was, but I didn't start until his second day in the hospital. Was that it, was it too late? Or was it digitalis toxicit? My God, I started him on dig for the atrial fib—not a high dose, but could he have had some metabolic problem and developed a really high level? Or did he have a massive heart attack that I should have foreseen, linked to his a-fib, or some other rhythm problem that we could have diagnosed and treated?

I run feverishly through one scenario after the next. What could I have done? What could I have failed to do? . . .

FOR THE NEXT few days I can't sleep, I stop eating, I can't pay attention to anything. I am obsessed by each detail of my other patients' care—could this person die suddenly overnight, too? What might I be missing? What might I be doing wrong? At the same time, I am hopelessly distracted. My own nebulous guilt hangs heavily on my shoulders, its weight almost unbearable. I'm terrified without being able to define why. Part of me believes that this is the end of my medical career, that I will be exposed as a dangerous idiot and a fraud, that I will lose my job, my prospects, everything I've worked for all these years. Part of me is simply paralyzed at the moral and ethical and existential horror of having perhaps killed someone. How would I be able to live with myself? This is a fear I have carried on some level from the beginning of my training in medicine, but now it crashes full force over me. It's one thing to think: I carry the responsibility for people's lives. It's another thing to be faced with the prospect of having betrayed that.

MY FRIENDS TRY to console me, to shake me back into reality. "If he was all that healthy, he wouldn't have been in the hospital," one says flatly. "Besides, when you're eighty, it's okay to just drop dead. You're entitled."

But nothing can calm me until I know. I wait for the autopsy results with my heart in my throat, half terrified that it will reveal some catastrophic error of mine for all the world to see, but mostly just needing to know, to have it over, to be done with this agonizing suspense.

It takes them two days to perform the postmortem, then—infuriatingly—the pathologist who did it goes to a conference, and no one can find his notes. The secretary tells me to call back the next day, Friday, which happens to be my day off. I think about going in, but it's summer, beautifully sunny outside, and I remind myself that no purpose would be served by my showing up at the hospital at this point. Whatever damage has been done, is done.

So I don't go in, but I call for the results. I talk to the Path secretary a half dozen times. The pathologist is in a conference, then doing an emergency frozen section for the surgeons, then at lunch. I had planned to spend the day kayaking and finally I realize that I can't put it off any longer if I'm going to go. I'll work through the weekend, but the pathologists won't. I can't wait until Monday for my answer. I end up at a pay phone, in a swimsuit, with my kayak waiting on the beach when I finally reach the pathologist.

"This is Dr. Transue," I say in my most severe voice. I am just able to be amused at the incongruity between the carefree, sunburned, swimsuited kayaker I must look like, the quaking guiltridden basket case I am inside, and the calm, serious physician I am trying to project into the phone.

"I'm trying to find out the postmortem results on Mr. Jamison." I look around, wondering if anyone can hear me.

The pathologist clears his throat. "Well." I expect, based on my experience of the last few days, some further explanation of delay, some excuse. We can't give you any information about that because... But instead he says, "What is it that you want to know?"

I wasn't expecting this. "Er . . ." I stumble. "Cause of death?"

"We didn't find a cause of death."

I absorb this for a second, confused. Please, God, don't tell me that after all this, there isn't going to be an answer. I don't think I could bear that.

"We're never going to find a cause of death. We can't. Mr. Jamison died of some kind of a cardiac rhythm disturbance. Most people do. I can't tell you exactly what caused that. Nobody can."

"Oh," I say meekly.

He clears his throat again. Having given what I later realize is his standard riff on "causes of death" to any clinician bold enough to demand one, he softens.

"I can tell you what he had," he adds, as if as an afterthought.

"Yes?" I say, almost without hope at this point.

"What he had," he says, "was metastatic lung cancer."

I barely hear anything more. It was everywhere, he tells me, his voice seeming to come from very far away. It was all over his lungs, his liver, many tiny metastases elsewhere. It was studding the sac around his heart, probably invading the nerves, which, he grudgingly accedes, was most likely what directly killed him. It might have been the cause of his a-fib as well, but it hardly matters. Even if we'd known the diagnosis from the beginning, there wouldn't have been anything we could do. I remember his chest X-ray on admission, completely normal; the cancer was growing in a diffuse pattern, hard to see, not in big nodules, the pathologist says. It isn't surprising that we didn't find it.

I feel as if a terrible sentence placed on me has been commuted. *I didn't do it.* His death was not my fault.

Perhaps it shouldn't matter, surely not this much. The essential fact of his death is unchanged. Knowing I am not to blame does not bring him back to life. And more than that, this telephone call does not change my worth or my skill as a physician. I am as careful and as fallible as I was an hour ago. I will still do my best, and I will still make mistakes, and someday I, like every doctor, will probably be responsible for some terrible error. The details of this one man's death do not change that. However it may feel, I would not have been a worse doctor if he had died from something I could have prevented, nor am I a better doctor because he didn't.

Even as I tell myself these things, the terrible tension that had knotted me up for these few days is relaxing, letting go.

I hang up the phone and go back to my kayak. The day is beautiful. I am young; my life, unruined, is ahead of me; and suddenly I remember that it's my day off, that it's okay to be a carefree kayaker as well as a physician. I look around and see the sunshine for the first time since Mr. Jamison died, feel it warming my face and arms. I have not killed anyone. I am not a terrible or a dangerous or a stupid person.

As I paddle onto the lake, I feel a dull ache of sadness at Mr. Jamison's death. Relieved of wondering whether I killed him, I can now wonder instead what will become of his wife, whether I could have better eased the loneliness of his last days. These are sorrows I can accept, I decide, rocked by the water underneath me. If and when I have worse things to live with, I will find a way. But for today, this is enough.

24. Teaching

The only thing stranger than not being an intern anymore is being in charge of one.

My month on Cardiology, an unusual service with only second-year residents, made a nice transition. I had a month with only the attending to supervise me, and no one for me to supervise.

The next month I was back on the wards at the county hospital, heading a team of my own. "My team": the words accurately express the possessiveness of it. My team. My interns, my students, my patients.

There's a strong argument that the transition from being an intern to a second-year resident is harder than the one from a med student to an intern. The latter is a transition to having power: as an intern you can write orders, give medications, request tests. But as a resident, in much deeper ways, you have responsibility. You supervise every decision that the intern makes, on a very specific level if you don't fully trust the intern, or a broader one if you do. The intern gathers the information, talks to and examines the patient, gathers the lab results; the resident is in charge of building all that information into an overarching assessment and plan. Of course, you sometimes do that as an intern, but you always know there's someone above you thinking through things, working them out. As a resident, you are the decision maker.

Also, the resident sets the tone for the team. You can't control whether it will be busy or slow, crisis packed or sleepy, but you determine how you, and your team, will react to each of those. Leading a team, I quickly realize, is partly about acting. An intern who's having a crummy day can stomp and sulk, and as long as the work gets done it doesn't really matter. A resident who does that will poison the spirit of the whole team.

I READ SO much in the mirror of my interns' faces—are they frightened? Do they feel supported? Do they have confidence in me? I'm always amazed that they don't feel a need to reassure me, as I try to reassure them, after a crisis. Can't they see my inner shaking? Don't they know?

"Okay, that's enough of those for today," I say, after our second code one evening.

"Don't you like codes?" my intern asks.

"No," I say.

"Really?" He sounds startled. "But you always seem so comfortable. Mellow."

"Really." I'm amazed. How could he not know, after all the times we've done this, how my heart sinks and my stomach lurches when the code pager goes off?

It makes me wonder about the residents I had when I was an intern, who seemed uniformly so cool and collected in a crisis, so unperturbed. What were they hiding, what were they feeling inside? I had more faith in some than others; what made the difference?

ONE OF MY first interns is very bright and very confident. Whenever I tell him something, he nods quickly, almost dismissively, as if to say he already knew.

I'm writing a note one night while he answers phone calls across the table. "There's this cross-cover guy," he says, looking up from the phone. "He's not doing well. I'm on my way to see him."

"Do you want me to come with you?"

"Yes."

I never thought I'd hear him say that. This brash young man, half a head taller than me and incidentally a few years older, usually seems to think that supervision is a hindrance. And now he's asking me for help.

His patient has heart failure and emphysema and has taken a sudden turn for the worse. We quickly examine him and review his information. "What are your thoughts?" I ask my intern.

"It could be a pulmonary embolus," he says. "Or a pneumonia."

"It could," I agree. "Although he doesn't have a fever and his heart rate's slow. Other ideas?"

"MI?"

"Always important to think about," I agree. "Anything else?"

He gives a deer in the headlights look.

"Sometimes we give these guys too much oxygen," I say. "If they're not used to it, the higher blood oxygen levels can suppress the respiratory drive, and then their carbon dioxide levels go up, and that shuts the brain down."

He nods.

"Okay, that's a good list. Now, what shall we do?"

"A chest X-ray, an EKG, an ABG?"

"Fabulous."

We send a nurse to order the X-ray and the EKG, and my intern runs off to get materials for the ABG, or arterial blood gas. It's not a hard procedure. You need blood from an artery to analyze levels of oxygen and carbon dioxide, and acid-base balance. The easiest place to get it is the radial artery in the wrist. With a special syringe and a tiny needle you push into the pulse—coming at it from a forty-five-degree angle is best—until the arterial blood shoots into the syringe, propelled by its own pressure.

My intern is swabbing the patient's wrist with alcohol, syringe in hand. I always liked doing ABGs, the feel of the pulse, the redness of the blood as it fills the syringe. I realize with a stab of jealousy that, as the senior person on the team, I'm not supposed to do them anymore.

Maybe he'll miss it, I think, with guilty hopefulness. Of course, he never misses anything, he's Mr. Confidence.

But he does miss it. The nurse is hovering, wanting to try next, and I think, no fair! It's my turn. But I'm supposed to be supervising.

The nurse pokes for a while at the patient's wrist and then withdraws the needle, looking frustrated. Then a magical thing happens: they turn to me. Both the nurse and the intern quietly turn to me. Of course, I remind myself, I am the senior resident. I pull on gloves and take the needle, feel the pulse. It's bounding, and I laugh with pleasure at the vehemence of that life force. "Don't laugh until you see how hard it is," the nurse says darkly, misinterpreting. A second later the bright red blood is gushing out into my tube, steady and reassuring. I smile at the familiar but still powerful thrill of it, to tap blood out of someone's artery. My intern breathes softly in admiration, "You da woman." I shake my head.

That tube will give us our answers, along with the normal EKG and chest X-ray. His oxygen is too high, his carbon dioxide is rising, and just turning down his oxygen will bring him back to normal.

The nurse is on the phone saying, "Your husband is having some trouble, let me have you talk to the doctor." I've only just slid the needle out of the man's arm when I realize that the phone is being held out to me. The intern takes the vial of blood and reaches to hold pressure on the patient's arm, another quiet gesture of respect, as I strip off my gloves and reach for the phone. I hold my hand over the receiver and ask for the one thing I don't know about him. "What's his name?"

"Wilson," the nurse and intern say together. "Peter Wilson."

I nod, lift the phone to my ear. "Mrs. Wilson, this is Dr. Transue. . . ."

25. Ashley and Alexa

My first introduction to Ashley was in my month as an intern in the ICU. She'd been admitted the night before to one of the other interns, and I listened on morning rounds as he presented her story.

"This is a thirty-two-year-old female with end-stage liver disease secondary to alcoholic cirrhosis. She came in last night with a variceal bleed, got transfused eight units in the ER. GI went down with a scope but couldn't see anything but blood. She lost her airway, had to be put on the vent. On admission to the ICU . . ."

As he launches into her vital signs, I turn to study her, lying in the bed. Her skin is a strange ashen yellow color, a product of anemia and jaundice. It's an alien color, not a hue that human skin should have, as if she were being shown on a video screen with the color wrong. Her arms and legs are emaciated, her belly round and protuberant with the pregnant appearance of severe ascites. She's lying extremely still—sedated, I assume—looking very small and frail in the large ICU bed. She's on a ventilator, and her chest rises and falls in a steady rhythm. The tube down her throat and the tape which secures it keep me from getting a clear sense of her face; I can see her sunken temples, her protruding cheekbones. And her left eye, swollen shut in an enormous knot of blackened purple-green.

The next night I'm on call, and a nurse pages me in the late evening to say that Ashley's husband is there and wants to talk to a doctor. I give him a brief summary of what we've done.

"Will she be okay?" he asks, his eyes dark, unreadable.

"I don't know," I say.

"I found her in a pool of blood," he says. "I know her liver's bad—she knows it, too. But she keeps drinking."

He looks at me as if for an answer. A thousand thoughts and questions are in my head, about the black eye, about why she drinks, about what she's doing to herself and what he's doing to her. But no words come.

"She's pretty sick," he says uncertainly.

"Yes," I say.

"Will she be okay?" he asks again.

"I don't know," I repeat.

After he goes, I go to her bedside and stand, watching her quietly, for several minutes. She's still on the ventilator, a still, yellow shape in the middle of the bed. Some splash of bright color catches my eye amidst the white sheets and yellow skin. I look down and realize she has chipped, bright pink nail polish on her emaciated yellow fingers.

She made it through that episode, went home. Not long after that I admitted her again, this time on the general medical ward. She'd broken her leg and the orthopedists were afraid she might go into alcohol withdrawal, so she came to my team. The black eye had faded, but there were new bruises. She'd given three different stories about how she'd broken her leg.

Her nails were lavender now. Her hair was thin, falling out from malnutrition, but she tied what there was in a ponytail at the top of her head, cheerleader style. She spoke breathlessly in a little-girl voice.

"You are so sweet to keep checking on me," she said.

"I like checking on you," I said. "But don't give me too much credit, it is my job. . . ."

"You're a cutie," she said.

Everyone was a cutie or a sweetie or a pumpkin. "Ashley," I said. "We need to talk."

She smiled brightly. She'd done her mouth in pink lipstick this morning. Pink lips, lavender nails, blue eyelids, yellow skin and eyes. The contrast between her little-girl style and her dying woman's body was so glaring I could barely look at her. "What do you want to talk about?" Her tone suggested I might want to play word games or discuss boy bands.

"I want to talk about your bruises and your black eye and how you broke your leg."

She smiled at me forgivingly. "Oh, you're like the others. You think it's Samuel. But you don't understand, Samuel would never hurt me."

Samuel was the boyfriend, or maybe husband—she introduced him different ways at different times. The father of her two children. He came to see her sometimes but avoided the medical staff. I probably should have tried harder to see him, but actually I was just as glad he stayed away. I wasn't sure I could be civil.

"Does someone else hurt you, then?"

She laughed a high, tinkling laugh. "Of course not, silly! Nobody would hurt me."

"Ashley, I know you don't want to talk about this, and I can think of any number of good reasons why. I'm not going to do anything or talk to anyone without your consent. I couldn't, even if I wanted to. But you need help, and I can't help unless you talk to me."

"You're so sweet." She smiled a glittery smile. "Worrying your head about me when you've got so many things to think about. But please don't."

I tried a different tack. "You told the medics you fell down the stairs, you told the ER you tripped on a curb, and you told me you slipped on a rug at home and fell over the sofa. Why do you have three stories, if you aren't trying to hide something?"

"I'm absentminded, I get confused." She smiled. "But really. Nobody would ever hurt me."

Defeated, I offered one final try. "If you ever change your mind, I'll always be ready to talk, okay?"

"How can I change my mind when there's nothing wrong?"

My resident, my attending, and the social workers had no better luck. Soon she was well enough to go home. I went over her medicines with her before she left.

"We'll get you a supply of the medicines for your liver, and your iron, to last until you see your clinic doctor."

She nods.

"You've been taking oxycodone for your pain, and I know you have a bunch of those at home."

She frowns. "No, there aren't any," she says.

I frown, looking at the pharmacy record in my hands. "It says here you got fifty of them three days before you came in."

She hastens to explain. "Samuel flushed them down the toilet. He said he didn't want me taking those things, so he took them away."

I nod slowly. Yeah, Samuel seems like the type to flush a perfectly good bottle of narcotics down the toilet. Is he taking them, or selling them? I wonder cynically.

"We'll give you a few more," I say. "You can come to clinic and get a few days' supply at a time. In the future," I add, as if there were any point, "it would be better for Samuel to bring medications you're not using back to the clinic, instead of flushing them down the toilet. It's important for us to be able to keep an eye on things."

"Sure," she says brightly.

HER PRIMARY CARE doctor works in my clinic, and on her next visit Ashley stops in to see me. She pokes her head in the doctors' workroom door.

"Dr. Transue!" Her face lights up and she reaches out with both arms to hug me. She looks a little worse, her belly still more bloated and her face still more gaunt, her makeup thereby more garish in its contrasts.

"I'm doing great," she gushes. "Just great. The kids are terrific, Samuel is great, he's taking care of me—"

Her voice is high and breathless, lisping slightly. She beams through her sunken face and yellow eyes—at least neither of them is black this time. She clings to my hand as she talks.

I have a flash of unexpected anger. You are an adult woman, I want to say. You are the mother of two children who are going to have to grow up without you. And you are here through choices you have made, as well as stars that have been aligned against you. Just once, before it's too late, acknowledge the reality of what is happening. You are going to die! We know it, and you know it. So die as a grown-up, not as a child. . . .

THE NEXT TIME I admitted her was in my second year. I had just started on the medical wards, heading a team with two interns. One of them was Alexa Williams, an incredibly smart and empathetic intern with whom I loved working. We shared a birthday and a sense of humor.

My breath caught when the ER doc gave me Ashley's name. "I guess she's been in a lot," he said. "This time it's encephalopathy. Her liver's getting worse, her ammonia level is through the roof, and she's confused."

Alexa and I went down to admit her. Ashley didn't recognize me. She seemed to be disintegrating before my eyes. I fought back tears.

Our next admission that night was a thirty-nine-year-old with metastatic ovarian cancer. I took care of her without the interns, since they were busy and it was clear she wouldn't be with us long. She came in from a nursing home to die, and she did, at around four in the morning, with her ten-year-old daughter and her sixty-year-old mother in the room. They all tried so hard to be brave.

ASHLEY NEEDED INTRAVENOUS medication and fluids, but no one could get an IV into her ravaged veins. "We'll need to do a central line," Alexa reported.

"What kind do you want to do?" I asked.

"Let's do a femoral."

I'd gotten comfortable with femoral lines over the last year. I nodded. "Call me when you're ready."

She calls me into the room a few minutes later. I lean over Ashley, who is drugged out on her body's own ammonia, which her liver can't clear.

"Ashley, sweetie, we just need to pop a little IV in your groin."

She mumbles incoherently.

I shake her awake. "Is that okay?"

"Fine," she says, before drifting off again.

I've gotten consent from her husband and her mother. Nobody is sure whether they're really married, and who is the legal decision maker when she's too out of it to choose. The hospital ethics team is sorting it out, and in the meantime I'm hedging my bets by checking with both of them. Luckily, so far, they've agreed.

Alexa, in sterile garb, unwraps the central line. It's about six inches long and the diameter of a telephone cord. We stare at it for a moment with the same thought.

"Did you just say, 'We're going to pop a little IV in your groin?'" she whispers.

"Yep." We both stare at the thick cord of the line in front of us, and at the pile of implements involved in putting it in. She titters and then I titter, and we both have to pause to gain our composure before we get started. Luckily, in the interim, Ashley has fallen asleep, and she continues to snore quietly while we work on the line.

Later we will tell the story to the other intern, and Alexa and I will both be in stitches on the floor: "Pop in a little IV . . ." We will laugh hysterically at the depth of my understatement, at my desperate cheeriness in the face of tragedy.

ALSO THAT NIGHT we admitted two drug users with abscesses, another with endocarditis, three homeless men with pneumonia, a young man with unexplained kidney failure, an older woman with a blood clot in her legs, three people with drug overdoses, two deliberate and one not, two people in alcohol withdrawal, and one old man whose family dropped him at the entrance of the ER because they didn't want to take care of him anymore. Plus Ashley and the dying woman. I counted how many of these I could truly help. Maybe two, I thought. Maybe the kidney failure and the blood clot. Two out of sixteen.

THE NEXT DAY seemed endless. There were procedures to be done, notes to write, discharge arrangements to be made. I was there until 8:00 P.M. without a pause except to gobble food and go to the bathroom.

When it was finally time to leave, I stepped out the hospital's double doors in a daze. The sun was just about to set. The water of Puget Sound was lit a gorgeous silvery blue, and the snow-capped Olympic Mountains were silhouetted against the flaming sky. The lights of the waterfront glittered, and a few stars were coming out overhead.

I sat down on the hospital steps, overwhelmed. How could such beauty coexist in the world with everything I had just seen? I sat and stared as the red sky deepened and the stars brightened overhead. As the last sliver of the sun slipped past the horizon, I began to cry.

"Beautiful, isn't it?" said a voice behind me. It was Alexa.

I hastily wiped my eyes, not soon enough. "Oh—" she said.

"I'm okay," I said. "Just overwhelmed."

She nodded. "I was wondering if that feeling eventually went away. I guess I'm glad it doesn't."

I shook my head ruefully. "For better or worse, no."

We looked at the fading sky together. "How can it be so beautiful?" she asked.

"I don't know," I said.

ASHLEY DIED A month later. I ran into her clinic doctor. "You heard about Ashley?"

"No," I said. "I hadn't."

"I'm sorry," he said. "I meant to tell you. It was a week or so ago. She bled. . . . It was quick. She didn't suffer."

I nodded.

"I'm surprised she made it this long, really," he said gently.

"I suppose I am, too."

I told Alexa. She nodded slowly. Both of our eyes went wet, and we sat for a long time in silence. It only occurred to me at that moment that Ashley, Alexa, and I were within a few years of the same age.

26. TTP

There are certain diseases that internists love. They tend to be rare disorders with complex consequences, difficult to diagnose, important to treat. Diagnoses that make us feel clever, for finding them, and powerful, for treating them. Pheochromocytoma and carcinoid, obscure endocrine tumors with strange and varied effects. Immune system disorders like scleroderma and familial Mediterranean fever. And thrombophilic thrombocytopenic purpura, or TTP, a disorder that affects the kidneys, the platelets, and the red blood cells, and leads to mental confusion, rashes, blood clots, and excessive bleeding. It's treated with plasmapheresis: drawing out the patient's blood, filtering out the plasma, and replacing it with new plasma. Obviously you can't remove too much blood at once, so it's done in a continuous cycle, with blood being simultaneously removed and put back in.

More is understood about TTP today than when I was a resident, though even now it has a certain mystery about it. It generally affects healthy young people, and can bring them from perfect health to the point of death in only a few weeks or days.

JILLIAN WAS A healthy young person. She didn't think about doctors much; she saw one every few years for a Pap smear. She had a part-time job at a bakery with no health insurance, a nice boyfriend, a cheerful outlook on life. When the rash appeared on her legs she ignored it for a few days, even as it started to grow, raised purple dots and tiny flat red ones starting on her ankles and climbing up her thighs. Over the next few days she got tired and pale. Her boyfriend worried, but it wasn't until she stopped midsentence in a conversation and couldn't go on that he swept her into the car and brought her to the ER.

I was leading a ward team, still with Alexa as my intern. The ER called to say they were admitting someone with anemia and a rash. They were very busy and didn't have time to wait for the rest of her labs, but clearly she needed to come in.

We examined her in the ER. Alexa started writing her admitting orders while I pulled her labs up on the computer. "Damn," I whispered. "I think she might have TTP."

She set the orders aside and read over my shoulder. "What do you do for that?"

"Steroids," I said. "And plasmapheresis I think. We'll call Hematology, they'll know."

"How long does it take to improve?"

"Hell if I know. I've never seen it before."

ONE OF THE roles of a resident is to go to a daily conference called residents' report. After rounds, the interns go off to get work done and the residents gather to present and discuss their interesting cases. I was a little intimidated by residents' report during this month. There was one other second-year resident leading a team, but mostly it was third-years, and a particularly brash and confident set. They would discuss the minutiae of recent research on some rare thing that had come up in the Intensive Care Unit, while my fellow second-year and I looked at our watches and wished we could get back to work. Our cases seemed bland and trivial by comparison, our concerns small-minded: how to take care of our patients, not what theories might someday shed light on them. I felt stupid then, for not knowing what the residents ahead of me knew, for not having all the latest studies at my fingertips. A year later I would understand I had been fine all along. It takes time to settle into the basics when you are first leading a team, and only when you're comfortable with these do you move to the next level. A second-year isn't supposed to know everything a third-year knows.

The day after Jillian came in I practically skipped into resident's report. I had a case! A wonderful, interesting case. I cleared my throat for attention at the beginning of conference. My voice wavered at first, unused to offering anything but a quiet suggestion in this room. But then it steadied. The residents quieted as my story began to unfold. After I described her exam—that lovely rash!—we paused so everyone could offer ideas and theories. Then the room went quiet as I recited her strikingly abnormal lab values, her almost absent platelets, her fragmented blood cells, her kidney failure. Excited murmurings went up around the table. Could it be anything else? Or was it TTP?

It was, indeed. The hematologists came and made thorough recommendations. "The next few days will be critical," the hematology fellow said. "Either she'll turn around, or . . ."

For the next few days we hovered over her like hawks. Her labs were drawn three times a day and we waited for them as if for lottery numbers. Clinically, she stayed about the same, though her confusion lifted. Her numbers stayed steady, surely a good sign, we thought. Then, on the third day, her labs improved. She was out of the woods. Now it would be a slow, steady recovery.

*   *   *

TTP WASN'T ENTIRELY unheard of; the hospital saw about one case a year. Still, Jillian was a feather in my cap, my personal claim to fame. People stopped me in the hallway to ask how my TTP person was doing. "Great," I would say, taking absurd pride in the fact, though most of the work was my intern's and most of the decision making was the hematologist's. Still, I had a sense of propriety; it was my team, and she was my patient.

Jillian, meanwhile, was a delight. She was always cheerful, always glad to see the team. Alexa, as her intern, spent the most time with her, prerounding in the morning and checking in with little things; they connected well, and I enjoyed watching them, seeing Alexa grow into her role as a young doctor, seeing Jillian's confidence in her.

Jillian's boyfriend brought huge boxes of brownies from the bakery where she worked, thick heavy brownies laced with chocolate or caramel. She expressed surprise one day at how friendly everyone was, and we didn't have the heart to point out that three of our patients had sworn at us on rounds that morning, and one had overdosed in his bed on heroin brought in by a friend, then spat and cursed when we resuscitated him. Jillian's calm, quiet room and her ever-ready smile, not to mention the supply of heavenly chocolate, were an oasis in the grim desert of the hospital.

SHE'D BEEN PUT in an isolation room; meningococcal sepsis, a highly contagious and dangerous disease, can cause some similar findings to TTP, so we had to take precautions until this possibility was eliminated. Her room had a little antechamber where staff could wash their hands and put on gloves and where, while isolation was in effect, a sealed door would keep air from escaping from her room. Once the isolation was discontinued, the door to the little room stayed open and gave the place an air of formality, like a little suite.

"I love this room," she said. "With its little antechamber. It's like a cabana. I keep wanting to say, 'Send in the cabana boy!'"

Taking the joke one step further, I said, "'No, um, the *other* cabana boy . . .'"

Everyone giggled, and Jillian looked up at me.

"You made a joke."

"Is that so strange?"

"I've never seen you laugh before. You always seem so serious."

She spoke without irony, and I was stricken. Had I become so concerned about my supervising role that I had lost my sense of humor? To my relief, however, the comment sent my team into gales of laughter. Things couldn't be too bad, I decided.

FINALLY SHE WAS well enough to go home. We gathered in her room for a last box of brownies and good-byes. Alexa came out a little after the rest of us.

"She's going to follow up with me in clinic!" she said exultantly. "I get to be her doctor!"

"Of course you do," I said, smiling. I'd waited to see if they would figure this out, or if I would need to suggest it. "How wonderful for both of you."

A year ago I would have been the one who was closer to her, the one she would have picked to be her doctor. I suppress a twinge of envy, and settle for being proud and glad for both of them.

27. Covered in Bugs

The call from the ER begins with the words: "I'm sorry. . . ."

I smile, although there hasn't been much to smile about today. I'm working at the county hospital now. It's been busy, though who am I kidding, it's always busy. This ER doc is a friend of mine, and it's good to hear her voice.

"It's okay," I say. "Whatever it is." I pull out another card to add to my already thick pile of patient sheets.

"We've got this guy for you who's covered in bugs."

I write down "covered in bugs" on the card, and wait for more.

"I think he's got some cellulitis around some of the bites," she says. "It's a little hard to see his skin right now."

"What kind of bugs?" Fleas, lice?

"A bunch of kinds."

"All right. Anything else?"

"That's it."

"Doesn't sound too bad," I say. All the complicated people I've gotten from the ER today, and they choose to apologize for this one?

"Wait till you see the bugs."

My intern is busy with another admission, so I go down to admit him. I pause in the doorway of his ER room. He's sitting quietly, crouched over in the bed. He wears a dirty yellow T-shirt and black pants under his hospital johnnie, a black wool cap on his head. I catch a glimpse of yellowish hair and a matted white beard. His arms are black with dirt and scabs, and even from the doorway I can see the bugs. Big ones, little ones, all shapes and sizes. They're crawling and jumping on his arms, his head, his back, even his shoes. They've invaded the clean blue-and-white surface of the hospital johnnie. I'm powerfully reminded of the Peanuts character Pigpen, always drawn in the middle of a whirling black cloud. This is precisely the same image.

I take an almost involuntary step back, wincing in spite of myself, in spite of all the gore I've gotten used to. Perhaps the most startling thing is how calm he is, sitting very still, apparently oblivious to being the focus point of a small entomological civilization. He gives no indication of even noticing the bugs.

I'm bracing myself for the inevitable step into the room when suddenly I am rescued—I can only use that word—by the tap of a nurses' aide on my shoulder. "Doc? I was just going in to clean him up. Should I wait till you've talked to him?"

"No," I say too quickly. "No, no, that's all right, you go ahead. I'll talk to him after."

IT WILL TAKE a day or two and many washings to completely eradicate the bugs. The first time I examine him, though the black living cloud is gone, a number of stragglers are still hopping up and down his arms. I try not to lean too close to the bed.

We go through the usual round of medical questions and arrive at the social ones.

"Where do you live?"

"Under the Fifty-ninth Street Bridge." He glances up at me with a fierce look, as if defying me to challenge this address.

"How long have you lived there?"

"Twenty, thirty years."

"Where do you eat?"

"Soup kitchens mostly. And I find things." In Dumpsters, I assume.

"Do you get a chance to bathe at all?"

"I wash once a week in Elliot Bay."

Elliot Bay. I've stood along its banks near the docks many times, looking down at the water. Beautiful in the light of sunset but hardly clean, oily with ship fuel and floating garbage. Not to mention bitter cold. I shiver for more than one reason at the thought of someone immersing himself in it. On the other hand, he must have really wanted to bathe, to brave that.

"Do you smoke?" I ask.

"No."

"Do you drink?"

"Nope."

"Did you ever?"

"Sure." He squints at me as if this were a stupid question.

"When did you quit?"

"Nine, ten years ago."

"Why?"

He glances up, as if appraising me, then shrugs. "No money."

"I guess that's as good a reason as any."

For a brief moment he grins.

After I've talked to him, my attending goes into the room to meet him and chat for a while. He comes out grinning broadly.

"That man is a gnome," he announces. "He's like a gnome from a fairy tale, living under the bridge. Can't you see him marching out with his staff, demanding tolls and asking riddles of anyone who wants to cross?"

I burst out laughing, because it is a perfect description. Especially now that he's been washed up, his white spun-cotton hair and wispy beard and mustache worthy of an expensive doll in a clove-scented collector's shop. His posture is endearingly hunched, his movements slightly exaggerated, his eyes bright but beady and suspicious. He is a bridge gnome, I agree. He could have stepped right out of a Disney movie.

ONCE HIS SKIN is clean, it becomes very clear that he has cellulitis—infection of the skin around the bites—along with deep ulcers at some of the bites, which will take some time to heal. The bites still itch, despite all our medications, and we work with the nurses to find creative measures to keep him from scratching. We wrap long white gauze strips around the itchy wounds on his arms to prevent him from touching them; light gloves shield his fingernails. All this helps some but not much.

The nurses cut his toenails, his hair, and his mustache and beard. I'm slightly disappointed by this last. Though he looks more presentable, I miss the ghostlike mouth, his upper lip disappearing into a fog of white wispy hair, his voice emerging from a dark opening in the white profusion—it seemed more befitting to a bridge gnome.

ON THE THIRD day of his admission, I come into his room to find him sitting up in bed, carefully plucking imaginary objects from the air around his arms. He looks up as I walk in.

"There's bugs on me," he says.

We wonder if he might be in alcohol withdrawal, but his level was zero when he came in and he sticks to his history of not having drunk in years. He refuses sedatives, becomes increasingly paranoid that we are trying to poison him with our medications. He continues to pick at the imaginary bugs.

We get a psychiatry consult, and they say that he's almost certainly schizophrenic. Since he refuses treatment and he's not an acute danger to himself or anyone else, there's nothing we can do. They offer him follow-up and he refuses.

When his wounds are well on the way to healing we discharge him to a respite bed, a place that houses the homeless while they're recovering from being ill. He says good-bye politely, though during the last few days he has been angry and unwilling to talk much, anxious to leave. I am not surprised to get the call from the respite facility saying that he never arrived. I knew he was going home to his bridge. I watch for him whenever I go by there, ready to be charged a toll or a question, wondering how long it took for the real bugs to return and ward off the imagined ones.

28. Adrift

The pilot was one of a great many patients we admitted one night from the ER, and not, on the surface of it, one of the more notable ones. He was an elderly homeless man, coming in with pneumonia. He also had some kind of chronic neurologic problem that affected his speech, that had been worked up before and found to be untreatable. It was hard to take his history, hard for him to answer questions.

"I have trouble—" He pauses, stumbles. ". . . Finding words," he finishes at last, with difficulty.

My intern and I stick with simple questions: Have you been having cough? Fever? He has trouble putting more than a few words together, but can answer with yesses and nos, and we get by okay. His story is clear-cut, the chest X-ray and labs clearly confirming his pneumonia. Satisfied, I write his admission orders and an admit note.

We start him on antibiotics, and his fever quickly dissipates, he breathes more easily. Over the next few days, it becomes clear that in addition to the word-finding problem, he has a mild dementia. He won't stay in his room. He wanders aimlessly around the ward, usually looking for a bathroom, though we keep explaining that there's one in his room. He keeps slipping out of his hospital johnnie and pants, apparently accidentally, then going in search of new ones. He wanders through the hallways half-naked, with his sheet wrapped around him like a toga. The nurses, not unreasonably, suggest restraints, soft loose ones to keep him in a chair. He disturbs the other patients with his wanderings and his nakedness, besides he might get lost, or wander into some other patient's room by mistake and frighten her.

I see their point yet am loath to tie him up; he seems so sweet and harmless. Sometimes I give in, sometimes I resist. His door is just across the hall from the doctors' workroom. When we leave him untied, I find myself caught in a frequent game of dashing out to catch him as he wanders, toga clad, into the hallway. I steer him back into his room. He's perfectly willing to stay there, he just forgets after a few minutes, and we repeat the escape and return again. I know this isn't a reasonable way of doing things, but I hate to restrain him.

ONE MORNING I flip through his old chart, something of an academic exercise in someone with a simple problem like uncomplicated pneumonia; I've already read the neurology notes, and I'm not likely to find much else that will affect what we do during this hospitalization. He'll be here for a day or two getting antibiotics, then out to a respite place until he's completely better. Nothing to it, from a medical point of view.

Since I have a quiet moment, I page aimlessly through the chart. He's had a few small skin cancers removed from his face, and something in the Dermatology note catches my eye. I cross the hallway to where he is sitting, for once, quietly on the bed.

"Hey," I say.

"Hey." He smiles at me.

"I read something interesting in your chart," I say.

"Really?"

"Yup."

"Oh."

"I read that you were in a plane crash. Back in '45."

"Oh," he says, surprise showing in both his face and voice. "Yes."

"And that you floated on a raft in the South Pacific for—how long?"

"Six weeks," he says.

"Your plane crashed?"

"Shot down."

"Who hit you?"

"Japs, I guess." He pauses. "Well—" he adds.

"Yes?"

"Hard to say really—all such a blur." It's the longest sentence I've yet heard him speak. But his eyes are getting bright and soft, and he continues. "Just fire and noise and explosions—"

He pauses.

"What happened next?"

"Then we were in the water. On the raft. Me and the captain." His voice has become dramatically stronger, less stumbling, more fluent.

A look of intense sadness crosses his face.

"The others—well, the flak and the crash and then, maybe some hit the water alive and then drowned. . . . There were just the two of us that made it, the captain and I."

"How did you eat?"

"Oh, we had provisions. On the raft. Lots of provisions—not very good, but enough, and God knows we were thankful for them. Water, too." He looks thoughtful. "There was enough on the raft for the whole crew, and it was just us two that made it."

I nod, acknowledging the mix of luck and loss.

"What did you do, all that time on the raft?

"Told stories, sang songs. Talked mostly."

"What did you talk about?"

"Everything you can think of. Girls, our families, school, religion . . ." His eyes go soft and distant. "Everything," he repeats.

"You drifted to land eventually?" I ask, when he does not continue.

"No—a boat picked us up. A sub."

"How did they find you?"

"That's what I asked them. When they picked us up, I said: How in the name of God did you ever find us?"

He pauses, then goes on. "And the sub guy said: they'd been having trouble with their—what's that thing? That you look with?" He twists his hand into a swan neck, rotates it around.

"Periscope?"

"Yes. Periscope. Anyway, they were having trouble with their periscope, and they finally get it fixed; and the guy says, I put the thing up, twirl it around, and the first thing I see is *your* ugly face!"

He laughs heartily. "Gave him quite a start I guess."

"Lucky for you," I say.

"Lucky for us," he agrees gravely.

"That's not the best of the story, though," he adds.

My pager beeps, and I reach to quiet it. "What's the best of the story?" Ten minutes ago, I wouldn't have believed he could tell even this much.

"Well, after they picked us up, they took us back to Pearl Harbor. And once we got there, they took us to the hospital, to have a full medical exam, be checked out after everything we'd been through."

"Of course," I say.

"And this doctor's having a look at us, giving us the whole once-over, you know. We were sunburnt something awful; my eyes were almost swollen shut. Not to mention we'd been pretty well scraped up in the crash of course."

I nod. My pager beeps again, insistently.

"But the doctor's just getting started on us when this sergeant barges in, from our regiment, you know. And he says: We've got to get them back to the carrier! Right off! We need 'em!

"And the doc says, Now hold on, I think they need a little R and R after everything they've been through. Three weeks, he says, three weeks at least on one of those floating palaces—you've heard of them? Where they used to send us for a break—gorgeous things, they were."

I nod.

"But the sergeant says, No way, they're gettin' their asses back on

155

that carrier by nightfall. Lieutenant's orders, no two ways around it. Men, he says, you're comin' with me.

"And that old doc, he looks at him. All this time he's been standing there all quiet. And then he reaches up—he's wearing a white coat, you know? So he reaches up and pulls back his coat, and there are the three stars across his collar—"

He looks up to make sure I appreciate the significance of this. "That doctor was a three-star general!

"If you coulda seen the look on that poor sergeant's face! 'Yessir. Three weeks, sir. I'll get right on it, sir. I'm sorry, sir. . . . ' And all the while he's saluting with both hands, back and forth, practically knocking his hat off from the force of it. 'I'm so sorry, sir. . . . '

"Best three weeks I ever spent," he says, "aboard that palace. But that moment was better than all of it. A general! And that poor saluting sergeant . . ."

He chuckles long and heartily. He's still laughing, sitting in his bed in his makeshift toga, as I, in equal measure grateful for the piece of his story that I've caught and sad for the many others that I know I'm missing, duck out of the room to answer the call of my pager.

29. Taking It

He was a new patient added to my clinic schedule at the end of the day. It was a Friday afternoon. I would be on call on the wards the next day. I hadn't done any of my paperwork yet, and it was already almost five o'clock.

"There was a scheduling mistake. He has an appointment, but there isn't anyone to see him—would you mind?" The clinic director smiles, and I glance away from him as I answer wearily, "Of course not." Does he have any idea, any memory, of what it's like to be an resident? To be always exhausted, always overworked and overtired, always having more to do than can be done? To carry more responsibility than you know enough to be comfortable with, to be drained and afraid all the time?

And then they take the one easiest day of the call cycle and add clinic to it. And when you think you're finally done—another hour of charts to do, then just enough time to have dinner, maybe catch a movie before going to bed early because you're precall—they throw on just one more. . . .

I fight back panic and self-pity. Well—I think, hope springing eternal—maybe he'll be simple.

I pick up his chart, flip to the problem list. "History of alcohol and drug abuse." And then the even more dreaded: "Chronic pain."

"Fuck!" Under my breath I curse the clinic director for doing this to me, the people at the front desk for screwing up the schedule, the patient for being there, myself for giving up my life to this entire, ridiculous, out-of-control business. I choke back the rush of tears that rises to my eyes. "Fuck everybody—"

The hot wave of anger and panic washes through and then past me. I will myself to calm, pat my hot eyes and forehead with my chronically cold fingers. I've been so tired for so long, sometimes I just don't know if I can take anymore.

Resolutely I pick up his chart.

He doesn't look the way I had expected. He's well put together, shabbily dressed but clean, his beard and mustache neatly trimmed. He doesn't have the shifty posture I anticipated, the furtive, despairing, desperate eyes. I chide myself for the stereotype, at the same time knowing that it was born from sad experience, not prejudice. I've seen a lot of despair and emptiness inside this room, much of it under the rubric of "drug abuse" and "chronic pain."

This man's eyes are clear, his posture at once confident and humble. He's here about the pain, he explains quietly, when I ask what brought him in today. He was, well, wild, in his young days, he explains, slightly inclining his graying head. He got thrown off one too many motorcycles, bruised up in one too many fights. He's got pins in his back and both legs from various orthopedic repairs, and the whole business just hurts.

He tells me all this matter-of-factly, without elaboration or much emotional display. The pain keeps him from work, from exercise. He tried to take classes to teach literacy, which is something he's always wanted to do—and which, he admits shyly, he thinks he'd have some talent at, "because of my experience." But he just couldn't sit in a chair that long because of the pain. He's taking huge amounts of Tylenol and ibuprofen, maximal doses of a new nonnarcotic analgesic, and daily oxycodone as well. All this keeps the pain livable but not really controlled.

My ears prick up at the mention of narcotics. This is the secret fear, difficult to escape with any chronic pain patient, but especially a known addict. The fear that they're using you, that their stories are just an elaborate ploy for a secondary gain. Medication seeking, like almost nothing else, poisons the doctor-patient interaction. When someone walks into your office you have to be able to assume that you share the common goal of making him healthy; whatever differences you may have about what that means or how he should get there, and whatever barriers may stand in its way, you share the goal, you have solid ground from which to work. Otherwise he wouldn't be there, right?

When you're holding the prescription pad and a patient is lusting for narcotics, all the rules change. Even just a year of residency has made me wary and suspicious when someone comes into my office and says he's taking chronic oxycodone. And yet, even though I go tense when he mentions it, I find myself trusting this particular man. I don't think he's pulling anything on me.

Once we've finished talking about his pain and reviewing his medical history, I go on to ask about smoking, alcohol, illicit drugs. He gave it all up two years ago, he says. Alcohol was the worst, his first and greatest downfall. The other drugs just went along with it and helped to ease his physical pain. It wasn't hard giving up cocaine or the occasional shot of heroin, but alcohol was the fiery demon in his breast. "So much I didn't know, then," he tells me, eyes suddenly focused far away, "about how much I was hiding from, how much I used alcohol to cover up all the difficult things in my life. Everything that was hard, painful, difficult—I used alcohol to take it all away. For a huge part of my life I did that. I never learned to deal with things, I never had to grow. So you can see how difficult it would be, to give it up and then realize that, on top of the thing itself, there was all this other work I had to do."

"How has it been since then?" I ask, when he comes to a stop.

"I do it day to day," he says. "Some of the days are hard, some easier. I go to meetings. I do my steps. I take it one day at a time." He gives a sad but resolute smile.

"The pain makes it harder, though. To have come so far, to have changed so much, and still be stuck with this—to know I'll always be stuck with this. Not—" He looks up suddenly, concern in his eyes. "Not that I'm complaining. It's my fault, I know that. I brought it on myself. I have no one else to blame. Still—to live with the pain, day in, day out, to imagine spending the rest of my life this way . . . just in pain, all the time . . ."

He pauses for a long time.

"I had this moment when I thought: 'I can't do this anymore. I'm on the point of giving up.'

"And then I thought about it, and I said: What does that mean? I mean, really. It's one thing to say, 'I'm going to give up,' but what would that be, what would that look like?

"And I thought, there's only a few things I can think of that giving up could be. One is to go back to drinking. And I'm not going to do that. That's over for me. That's just another way of dying, an ugly, undignified way, something less than human. About the only thing I know in life is that drinking isn't an option.

"And the other thing it could mean is—just not trying anymore. Not getting out of bed in the morning. Not making the effort.

"And I thought—well, that's not where I am at all! That's not what I want. . . ." He looks up at me. Though he's frowning, his face is full of energy. "So that's when I realized. I may feel like I can't take it, like I'm ready to give up. But the truth is, that's not it at all. That's just words—I can take it, I will go on. I just . . . don't quite know how yet."

His brows are furrowed in intense concentration. Suddenly he shakes his head.

"I'm sorry, Doctor, I'm just rambling. You don't need to hear any of this. It's just stuff I was thinking. . . . Does it make sense at all?"

"All the sense in the world," I say.

I WOULD LIKE to be able to say that I walked out of that room completely rejuvenated, counting my blessings. Ready to finish my charting, ready for call. I can't quite claim that. I was still tired, still weary and worn, if anything a little more drained from the conversation.

But I had reclaimed—rather, I had been given back—my focus, my perspective. I am tired, yes; fatigue is an occupational hazard of this profession, something I will not escape in residency at least. Though I will be tired, I don't have to be bitter. I can be angry at my field yet not be angry at my patients. And I will keep getting up in the morning, because even when I think I can't take it anymore, what else would there be to do?

30. Waiting for a Room

A small, eighty-five-year-old woman comes in to the ER with pneumonia. We are busy, and she clearly needs to be admitted, so I spend only a little time with her before sending her upstairs.

"It's all very well to be old if you're healthy," she says suddenly, as I am about to walk away.

"Yes," I agree.

"But if you're all falling apart, like I have been the last ten, fifteen years . . . what's the point?"

She shakes her head in disgust. She seems to be talking more to herself than me.

"You don't look like you're all falling apart," I say soothingly, trying to comfort her.

She shakes her head, dismissing this. "Unfortunately, it's not that you have much choice," she goes on. "I keep telling my daughter: what's this all about? What am I still doing here?

"And she says, 'God isn't ready for you yet. He hasn't got your room fixed up. He hasn't called you and you're just going to have to wait until he does.'"

"I see," I say, smiling at her.

A nurse walking by has overheard the exchange and grins at me. I shrug and smile back. "Housekeeping can get pretty backed up up there," I murmur as we walk down the hallway. "All those whites to keep clean."

"If it's such a problem here, why not there, too?" she answers. "'On earth as it is in heaven—'"

The old woman sits on a stretcher in the hallway for an hour, waiting for a room to be ready on the ward upstairs.

31. Broken Souls and Bodies

Halfway through a twelve-hour ER shift, a week into my month there, I find myself in Trauma Room 2, where the surgeons are playing a losing game of tug-of-war with death on a blood-drenched field.

The medics were still doing CPR as they brought him in the door. He'd had some kind of massive trauma, though I didn't hear the story. The surgeons pulled me in to run the code, so I, technically, am presiding over this drama. I'm not sure why. Usually the surgeons do these codes, but they asked me to run things from a medical perspective—drugs and shock and all that—while they try to assess and control the traumatic damage.

It sounds reasonable, but it's an odd position, since the two systems aren't totally independent and the surgeons keep doing things I don't expect or sometimes don't even know about. His abdomen has been cut open. All I see is a bloody mess in there, occasional recognizable bits of organ floating in a sea of blood. I'm not sure quite what they're doing, and I don't really have time to stop and ask.

"Continue CPR," I call out, after a pause to assess rhythm.

I look up and they're cutting his chest open with a saw.

"Okay, don't continue CPR, if you're going to do that," I murmur.

A moment later someone is doing cardiac massage, their hand inside his chest, squeezing the heart directly to make it pump.

"Do we have a femoral pulse with that?" I ask.

The surgical R3 looks up. "We cross-clamped the aorta."

I glance down into the open thoracic cavity where I can see only a pool of blood, trying to absorb this fact. "Cross-clamped the aorta." I experience a moment of pure absurdity. What are we doing here? What am I doing, trying to run a code without even knowing which major vessels we've got running, without knowing they'd cut off blood supply to everything from his waist down? What are they doing, opening the chest of a man we all know is going to die anyway, thinking they could save a man who needs to have his aorta cross-clamped? I see myself for an instant as a sort of crusty maiden aunt, complaining about the excesses of today's young. "Is that a *nice* thing to do?" I want to ask. "Is it civilized behavior to go around cross-clamping people's aortas?"

Instead I say, "Okay, do we have a carotid pulse?"

I CALL IN my attending, Alex, for backup. Rather than taking over the code, which I half hoped he'd do, he decides that the heart needs to be warmed. He sends students running for heated saline bottles. Then he pours them in a steady stream over the heart, mixing the free flow of blood in the room with an extra volume load of saline. The bloody water pools steadily in the sheets on the stretcher, then suddenly overflows, cascading in a broad red river down Alex's leg, soaking his pants, his shoes.

"Shit," he murmurs, and keeps pouring.

The code continues.

"Monitor shows an organized wide-complex ventricular rhythm," I say aloud in a pause in cardiac massage, partly for the code stenographer to record, partly because it's easier to think aloud. "Do we have a carotid pulse with that?"

"No," answers someone after a moment.

"Okay," I say. "So we're in PEA." Pulseless electrical activity: a rhythm on the monitor but no pulse. It used to be called EMD, electro-mechanical dissociation. The pacer system of the heart is firing but the muscle doesn't contract.

"Not exactly," points out Alex. He gestures, and I look down into the thorax at the heart, still twitching in a regular if not entirely organized way. Theoretically in EMD it would just be stunned.

"I'm really not used to having that kind of data," I say.

I stare the heart for a moment, waiting for a medication I've just ordered to be given.

"Well, continue cardiac massage—"

Then, miraculously, the heart's pulsation gets more organized. We stop compressions. "Carotid pulse?"

"Yes," announces a nurse, feeling his neck. "Thready, but yes."

"Blood pressure?"

"Seventy over forty," answers another nurse after a minute.

I look at the surgeons.

"We've got a rhythm, we've more or less got a pulse; let's go to the operating room. He's not going to get any better down here."

He's not going to get any better anywhere, I think.

"All right," I say.

They wheel him off down the hallway, blood sliding off the stretcher in a steady stream as they pass.

I watch the procession until it disappears into the elevator. I shake my head and frown, trying to collect my thoughts. I have a flashing memory of my first code, also in an ER. It was a simpler code than this, no blood and guts, no trauma; no staring at a throbbing, dying heart. I had no responsibility then, I did chest compressions but otherwise only watched. That day shook my world, and this strikes me mostly as just another messy piece of business. What's happened to me?

I was stressed but not scared when he came in, amazed but not thrilled that we got a pulse back, and would be neither surprised nor particularly upset to learn, a half hour later, that he'd died on the table in the OR. My heart rate never went up during the whole episode.

Telling the story later to a friend, I would be completely unable to answer her basic questions. How old was he? I never really even looked at his face. Was it a car accident? I assumed so—they usually are—but didn't know for sure. Was he drunk? What happened? Did he have family? I never thought to wonder.

I'm disturbed by my very imperturbability. How can I be so unfazed by this? Have I lost something, have I given up some essential part of my humanity, to see such a thing as this and not be moved?

I DON'T HAVE time to ponder long; patients have been piling up while we were busy in the code. I grab the next chart: a young man complaining of shortness of breath and "pain all over," according to the nursing note. Oh, joy, I think. Well, maybe I'll be lucky, and he'll have the flu or something.

I find him on a stretcher in the back hallway, a sign in itself that the nurses didn't feel he was particularly sick. It takes my eyes a second to adjust to him, after the bright lights and contrasts of Trauma 2. Everything about him—his clothes, his hair, his skin—is a uniform dark gray color, except for his bright blue irises and the whites of his eyes, peering startlingly out of the dark mass of the rest of him. He is, quite possibly, the dirtiest man I have ever seen. There are flakes of dirt and skin collecting in little piles on his sheet. I try not to breathe deeply but cough just from a whiff of the dust on him. He smells awful. The smell is familiar, and I finally place it. He smells like the monkeys I worked with years ago as an undergraduate. The smell of unwashed primate.

But there's something beyond dirt, something in his eyes, in the way he sits and the way he speaks; the distinct, indefinable but unmistakable aura of the mentally ill. I understand now why, despite a high-acuity complaint like "shortness of breath," he's sitting here in the back hall. We're not going to find anything—at least nothing we can treat here—and the triage nurses knew it.

Talking with him gets me no further, either medically or psychiatrically. I find nothing that points to a medical problem to account for his pain or his feeling of being unable to breathe. His thought and speech patterns are highly suggestive of schizophrenia, but he's not hearing voices or seeing things, he's not suicidal or thinking of killing anyone—nothing I could use to get him admitted to psychiatry.

I put on gloves before examining him. I don't usually wear gloves unless I'm doing something invasive or someone is bleeding. But he's just so filthy.

"Do you hurt here?" I ask, when I get to his belly exam. He's said he hurts everywhere else so far.

"Yes."

Thoughtfully, I palpate more deeply, looking for an area of localized tenderness.

"It hurts."

"I'm sorry."

I continue pressing, as gently as I can, trying to see if there's anything going on in his belly that we need to be worried about. Suddenly and roughly he shoves my hand away.

"I told you it hurts when you push, and you keep doing it!"

I stare at him in surprise, then turn stern for a moment. "I can't evaluate you without doing a thorough exam. I'll try to make it hurt as little as possible. But I can't help if I can't figure out what's going on."

"I'm sorry," he says, suddenly meek.

"That's okay," I say. "I'm sorry that it hurt. But I'm just trying to help."

He is quiet through the rest of the exam.

"I'm—I'm sorry I pushed your hand away."

"It's okay," I say. "I'm sorry that I hurt you."

I find nothing. The only thing wrong in his exam is that he complains of hurting everywhere I touch, and even there I can't find any of the qualities or patterns to the pain that would suggest a medical cause. He says he can't breathe—he tears up with fear telling me this—but not only do his lungs sound fine, he's breathing quite comfortably, not hyperventilating, not gasping, not using accessory muscles.

"How long has it been like this?" I ask.

"A long time."

"Days, weeks, months?"

"A long time."

"Months, do you think?"

"Doc," he says with sudden urgency, his eyes boring through me. "You've got to help me—"

I check his oxygen levels, a few basic labs, and a chest X-ray. I order an alcohol level and a drug screen, partly just to have something to do, to buy myself time. It'll take an hour or so for all that to get done, and in the meantime maybe I can think of something to do, or at least something to say to him.

THE TESTS, OF course, come back normal.

Armed with the normal results, I call the psychiatric social worker. I've done a medical workup and it's negative, so now the ball is in their court, right?

"I've got this guy here, came in with a complaint of pain all over and trouble breathing, but medically he's fine. I don't think he's a danger to himself or anyone else, but he's obviously got psych issues, and I was just wondering how that gets handled, whether there's a possibility you guys could see him."

"Is he suicidal? Is he homicidal?"

"No," I repeat patiently.

"Is he overtly psychotic? Is he grossly unable to care for himself?"

"I guess I'm not sure what that means," I say. "Do I think he's going to die tonight, no. Obviously he's not able to care for himself very well—"

"Just being homeless is not a reason for a psych eval," she snaps.

"I realize that," I say. "I'm quite sure that he's schizophrenic—"

"Is he hearing voices? Is he delusional?"

"He's not hearing voices. As for being delusional—well, he's got a delusion that he's suffocating when he's breathing fine, he's got a delusion of excruciating pain that I can't find a source for—"

"Just being schizophrenic is not a reason for an emergent psych eval," she says.

I want to say: Excuse me, what have I done to you? Why are you taking this tone with me? I'm tired, you're tired, we're all tired. We're all overworked and overwhelmed. But I'm just asking a simple question in an attempt to take care of my patient, and you're getting extremely hostile with me, and I don't understand. . . .

I'm just a little too tired to be confident that I could manage whatever confrontation might follow. So I let it go.

"He doesn't sound like someone we would see emergently," she says. "Get him an appointment and tell him to follow up."

"Thank you," I say stiffly.

I pour out my frustrations to the attending. "It sucks," she says. "But you've got to send him out."

I go back, stand beside his stretcher, at a loss for words.

"I know you hurt," I say, as gently as I can. "I know you feel like you're suffocating. But I'm afraid there isn't anything that we can do for you tonight."

He looks up at me with eyes that burn with agony.

"There are some doctors I think can help you, and I'm going to give you an appointment. But it will take a couple of weeks."

He closes his eyes.

"I—I'm sorry," I say.

"Hold my hand," he says suddenly. He stretches out a brown, crusted paw. I stare at it for a second. Then I reach out, and he takes my hand in his, clings to it as if for life.

After a minute I try to pull my hand away.

"Don't let go." He looks as if he were about to cry.

"Okay."

We stay like that for a long time, my hand clutched tightly in both of his, his eyes tightly closed. Finally he releases my hand. "I'll have the nurses get your things," I say quietly.

"Where are you going?" he calls as I turn to step away.

"There are other people I need to take care of."

"Oh."

I stare at him hopelessly. What am I supposed to do?

"Can I have some Seven-Up?" he asks meekly.

I'm so amazed at being presented with a need that I can fill that I'm almost confused for a moment. "Of course," I say, although I've told a half dozen other people tonight that I can't give them anything to eat or drink, that we have a policy of not doing that here, or, at best, that they'll have to ask their nurse. "We're an ER, not a cafeteria," I hear a dozen times a night. I go to the back room where we hide some 7-Up for patients who are hypoglycemic, fill a cup with ice and find a straw for him. His hands are shaking as he reaches for it.

He drinks half the cup, then looks at me in dismay. "I want to finish drinking it, but I can't set it down." I feel a spasm of irritation—I didn't go to medical school for this! But I get him an emesis basin to set down on the bed, which is stable enough to hold the cup.

"Thank you," he murmurs seriously.

I send a social worker to find him a shelter bed for the night, knowing how woefully inadequate this is. "I got him a place, but I doubt he'll stay," she says. Similarly, I press the appointment slip for Psychiatry urgently into his hand, having little faith that he'll get there.

I have to go see another patient and don't watch him as he leaves. But, continuing on through the busy night, I can't shake his image from my mind. His startling, bright eyes, shot through with inexplicable, unanswerable terror. The pressure of his hand clinging to mine, finally releasing me—I can only hope that he found something of use in that contact, some solace from his loneliness, a temporary salve for his inner demons.

I had a cousin who was schizophrenic, who spent a few years in and out of the medical and psychiatric system, and finally killed himself. He was younger than this man, and always had a home and was well cared for—in some ways—although obviously those advantages didn't save him. If he had lived longer might he have ended up like this, on a gurney in an ER someplace, begging for help. If so, would he have gotten better care than I gave this man tonight? Is there anything else I could have done? Would it have made a difference?

I continue working through the night, struggling with my own demons. But I am relieved, at least, to know I am still capable of being disturbed.

32. Conspirators

The ER charge nurse tosses me a chart.

"He's back." She rolls her eyes.

I've seen the name before, although I've never taken care of him. "What's his story?"

"Crotchety old bastard. Severe asthma and emphysema, still smokes, never takes his medicines. He lands here every week or so, not being able to breathe. He swears at the admitting staff, curses the nurses out—that kind of stuff."

I find him sitting up on the edge of his stretcher, gasping for breath and clinging to a tube which is pouring out a dose of aerosolized albuterol, a nebulizer, or neb for short. He has a long, white, dirty beard and matching hair, both flying in all directions. He wears a hospital johnnie and dirty gray-brown trousers.

He greets me with such a theatrical scowl that I grin before I can stop myself. For a moment I think this will be my worst mistake all day, then I realize it may be my best piece of luck. In response to my smile, I note some matching crinkle around his temples, a faint glimmer in his bright blue eyes.

"Good afternoon, sir," I say. I've noticed that though I don't call all male patients "sir," there's something about certain older men that just inspires it. "What can I do for you today?"

"Can't . . . breathe," he whispers, between drags on the neb. "Need"—he gestures to the machine—"this."

"Finish that," I say. "I'll come back."

His breathing improves after the neb and a shot of steroids. When he can breathe well enough to talk, he confesses his noncompliance to me cheerfully. "Probably I wouldn't feel so bad if I ever took my medicines."

"Why don't you?" I inquire.

" 'Cause I'm self-destructive." He looks up for a reaction. When I just smile, he shrugs. "Maybe just lazy."

"What can we do to make it easier for you?"

"Nothing. It's not you all. It's just me, I'm hopeless."

"Nobody's hopeless."

"I am," he says knowingly. He shakes his head. "Or maybe I like visiting you folks too much."

"That's probably it," I deadpan.

I leave him to work on a second neb. A few minutes later several trauma patients come in from a bad car accident, and all the nurses get tied up with helping them. He's due for a third neb. As I come down the hallway, I can hear him howling.

"I need another neb!" Just the fact that he can scream now indicates his breathing is better.

I poke my head in. "I understand that, sir," I say. "I'm trying to get someone to get you one. But all the nurses are busy just at the moment, and you want to know the truth?"

"What?" He looks at me suspiciously.

I drop my voice and whisper. "They don't teach us to do nebs in medical school."

"Really?" There's just a hint of a smile about him now.

"Really."

He thinks for a second. "It's easy," he offers. "You just have to squirt it in the bottom of the plastic thing." He holds up the latter for me to examine.

"Hm," I say.

He's watching me entreatingly.

"How about this," I say. "We'll try to figure it out. But you have to promise not to tell anybody, or I might get in trouble or something, okay?" This isn't true, of course, but . . .

"Okay," he says, granting me a conspiratorial grin.

Together we figure out how to open the plastic container, pour in a dose of albuterol, and start the air that drives the nebulizer. He puffs contentedly and waves me away.

By the end of his third neb, he's breathing comfortably, and his oxygen level is back to normal. This, and a round of steroids, is usually all he needs to get him through an episode. I make him a follow-up appointment we both know he won't keep, get him another set of the medications he never took before.

A few minutes later, I hear a small commotion from his room—he is refusing assistance in getting out of bed. After a moment he appears at the door, fully dressed in a filthy three-piece suit, cane in hand. With his tattered clothes and beard, his imperious manner, he has a sort of majestic shabbiness: an asthmatic modern-day King Lear.

He waves away the nurse at his shoulder, and points a wavering finger across the room toward me.

"The young doctor there will see me to the door," he announces in a loud, grand voice.

I look up, startled. Everyone turns to look at me, eyebrows high.

"Yes, sir," I say.

With all the gallantry I can muster, I stand and offer him my arm. He takes it more gallantly still, and we make our way slowly across the crowded ER to the exit.

33. How Old Are You?

I'm checking labs in the back room of the ER when one of the interns wanders by, looking for his resident. His name is Kevin. He's tall, handsome, cocky in an appealing way. I had a bit of a crush on him about six months ago, but then he grew a beard, which I hate, and he turned out to be obnoxious. I got over it.

Or so I thought. Now he's shaved, and he keeps dropping by the ER.

"Hey, babe," he says, coming up behind me and touching my shoulder.

"Hey, sweetie."

"How ya' doing?"

"Pretty well," I say automatically, then stop to consider the question more carefully. "Yeah, actually, pretty well."

He stands behind me as I study the computer screen and starts to rub my back. I close my eyes and relax into the pressure of his fingers. Damn, that feels good.

"Let's get married," I suggest.

He thinks a minute. "Okay," he says. Then he adds in a thoughtful tone, "One of the attendings was talking about her kids today. Having kids would be cool. . . ."

He holds me by the shoulders, and neither of us says anything. I find myself staring, unexpectedly, down a corridor of unrealized possibility. I've never so much as kissed this man. But there's no particular reason why Kevin and I couldn't get married, buy a house, have babies. Sure, we're not in love, don't really know each other—but people have done stranger things.

I shake off the vision, oddly vivid and slightly oppressive, of Kevin and a blond toddler and a renovated Victorian. I go back to copying down labs from the computer. He lets go of my shoulders.

One of the nurses walks by and tosses me a chart. "Real trip for you in six," she comments. I raise my eyebrows, but she just rolls her eyes and walks away. "He's got seizures," she comments over her shoulder. "You'll see for yourself," her tone suggests.

YOU LEARN TO be wary of "seizures," working in the ER. Some people really have them, of course, and a fair number of these end up in the ER at some time or another. There are also a lot of people who think they have seizures but actually have some other kind of spasm or shaking or dizziness, and others who have a psychiatric problem that manifests with seizurelike symptoms, called a conversion disorder. There are still others who pretend to have them for one reason or another—they're looking for benzodiazepines, a popular abuse drug used acutely for seizure control, or attention, or who knows what.

THE MAN IN room 6 is young, in his late twenties. A small guy with big eyes and thick glasses, he is perched cross-legged in the middle of the bed, with a funny half-frustrated, half-resigned look on his face.

He tells me his story. He starts with his list of antiseizure medications. He's on six, he says, and he lists out his doses—all at the upper limits of standard dosing. Despite all this, he has frequent episodes, and they've been happening even more often today than usual. He describes his "spells." First his arm feels weird, and then it lifts up or starts to twitch and wave. Sometimes it ends there, sometimes it proceeds to a full shaking spasm of his side. He's conscious through the whole thing, he says. Sometimes it starts with his leg instead, sometimes his other arm.

As he's talking, his right arm suddenly drifts into the air, then starts undulating. I think he's just demonstrating his typical symptoms, but he looks from the arm to me with a look of comical dismay. "There it goes again," he says.

He keeps talking, and after a minute the arm drifts quietly back into his lap.

There are certain things in a story that lead you to suspect someone isn't having true seizures. They don't sound quite right, don't fit the usual pattern and behavior of epilepsy. On some level, they just sound weird. On the other hand, there are rare but real forms of epilepsy that *are* weird—certain kinds of partial seizures, temporal lobe epilepsy and others, that have very strange effects. There's no real way, without an EEG, to know for sure.

There's an off chance the man is for real.

There are a few things I can do, labs I can check—electrolytes, drug levels, and so on—but I probably won't be able to sort out one way or another what's going on. That means I have to admit him. I have an unpleasant image of what it will be like calling the Neurology resident, the withering response I'll get: "You know this is bullshit. . . . Don't tell me you think seizure disorders look like this." But I want it to be real, partly because what to do will be simple, and partly because he doesn't feel crazy or fake to me.

I go to the computer system and pull up his records, hoping against all expectation and experience that there will be something useful there. Please . . . Please, let there be something.

And there, miraculously enough, it is. A clinic note from the neurologist. Three pages of evidence and detail. Complex partial seizures, documented by EEG, under moderate control on maximal drug therapy. The whole damned bizarre story is true.

I GO BACK in. "I saw Dr. Olson's note," I say casually, not sure if I want him to understand the significance of this—that I wasn't sure I believed him before, that now I do.

"Good," he says. There's a moment's pause. "That's a great notebook," he adds, pointing at the little green leather book I carry.

"Thank you," I say absently.

"No, really," he says.

I shoot him a quizzical look, and he looks down at his hands, as if apologetic for having spoken.

Beginning my neuro exam, I reach out a finger and move it through different areas of his gaze, testing his ocular motions. And then something odd happens. As you do the test, there's a point in the arc where the patient's line of vision intersects with yours. You, of course, are staring at their eyes, watching to see if they move properly. Occasionally, as this happens, the patient's focus will shift from your finger to your eyes. This is a basic animal reflex, to meet the eyes of someone who is looking at you. Normally, I just wiggle my finger and the patient's focus shifts back, and that's it. But this time, his glance shifts from my finger to my eyes and holds my gaze, for just a second, and then he grins.

And I, not knowing why, grin back.

He drops his eyes. "Sorry," he says.

"Everybody does that," I say dismissively, although I am distinctly and oddly shaken.

"You tricked me," he says. "Just kidding," he adds hastily. Then he blushes.

I suddenly realize that—I like this guy. With his funny little smile and his expressive eyes and his comic irritation at the whole circumstance. He's sweet.

*   *   *

I've understood since very early in my medical career that there's a certain chemistry to the doctor-patient relationship. There are people with whom you click, and people with whom you don't. With some people you feel a connection and communion immediately, and with others you have to fight to find it. With a few you never do. I've thought of it in relation to romantic chemistry, the nearest metaphor I could find.

The thing I'm feeling now isn't a doctor-patient click. It's a different click. It's feeling that if I met this guy at a party, I would give him my phone number. Nothing more or less than that. A blush, a smile, a sudden sense of vague disorientation. Nothing extreme, and yet it throws me completely, because I've never felt anything like this when talking to a patient before.

A patient.

You're not supposed to think these things about patients.

Sure, I've had patients who had crushes on me—this is part of the territory of being a young female doctor, of being any kind of doctor, I suppose. Occasionally it's offensive or annoying; usually it's not a big deal. You learn early on how to set clear limits, and few people try to cross them. I've even taken advantage of a crush once or twice. If a cajoling scold and smile from a "pretty young girl" will make an old man in clinic more likely to quit smoking, what does it hurt?

I've never returned a patient's crush before. I'm baffled by it, partly because he's such an unlikely romantic figure, this funny little man on the gurney, with his waving arms and too-wide eyes. He's not the kind of person to sweep you off your feet, not like the tall, handsome intern Kevin, for instance. Mostly I'm stunned, because I thought some magic power had come with my MD to deflect this sensation from anyone wearing a "patient" label. And I've just realized I was wrong.

Let me be clear that I was not confused about how to act: ignore it and then forget it. The situation was not complicated. I just hadn't believed I could feel this way, and I do.

"Dr. Emily," he says, reading off my name tag. There's a rule in this ER that we don't use our last names. It seems strange to me that the director should insist we use patients' last names but give out only our first ones—I understand it's some kind of precaution for our protection, but still.

"How old are you?" he asks.

"Old enough to be your doctor." This is my pat response.

"That's not an answer."

"It's all the answer I'm giving," I say. "When is your next appointment with Dr. Olson?"

I successfully distract him. As I'm walking out of his room a minute later, he calls back from the doorway: "You never answered my question!"

I shake my head and walk away.

I SEE TWO other patients while waiting for his lab results. When I return to his corridor, I find him standing in his doorway. He's captured a med student, and I catch a few words as I come around the corner: ". . . the tall, pretty one—" He breaks off as he sees me. "There she is!" The med student slips away, giving me a strange look.

"Are you married?" he asks.

"You know I'm not going to answer that."

"That's not too personal, is it?"

I don't answer.

"No ring," he points out. "But maybe you take it off to avoid tearing the gloves."

"Can we stick to questions about you?"

He looks pointedly at his empty fingers.

I can't help laughing. "I walked right into that, didn't I?"

"Married to a doctor—maybe a lawyer?"

I sigh.

"No, lawyers and doctors don't mix," he says. "A doctor, then, probably."

I shake my head.

*   *   *

"So I've got this guy who's having complex partial seizures," I begin. "Documented history, followed by Dr. Olson. Had a minor med change a couple days ago, and tonight he's—"

The attending's eyes are suddenly focused behind me and I look up to follow her gaze. A stretcher is being pushed toward us in the narrow hallway. We both step back into a nearby room to get out of its way.

"Go ahead," she says.

"Since seven P.M. he's been having a series of brief seizures, starting with his left upper extremity and proceeding—"

I break off as the stretcher goes by, pushed by a team of surgeons, headed toward the OR elevators. The body is draped in blankets, with only the head exposed. I see an endotracheal tube, attached to a bag which someone is pumping to ventilate him. The rest of the face is invisible under a wash of blood.

A thin, steady stream of blood is pouring from underneath the stretcher, leaving a red, puddling trail in its wake. A few feet behind the stretcher follows a volunteer, dressed in the hospital's hot-pink volunteer scrubs, waving a towel across the floor, mopping up the blood.

"Go on," says the attending.

"So, a series of partial complex seizures lasting thirty seconds to a minute and spaced a few minutes apart—"

I try to return to my presentation but break off again, to stare at the stretcher—now disappearing into the elevator—its pink-clad escort, and the red smear on the floor that will soon be the only sign of what just passed.

The attending is looking at me, waiting. I want to make a comment, but I can't think what there would be to say. "Sorry. Just having a little ER moment." She nods.

I go back into the seizure guy's room.

"I talked to the neurologists," I say. "They—and I—think you really need to come in to the hospital."

"When?" he asks.

"Now," I say.

"How about tomorrow?" he suggests.

"You've been having seizures all day. We don't know why they changed, and we don't know how they're going to keep changing. If you go home, they could start generalizing, and you could end up in status epilepticus. You could die."

"I think I'll be fine," he says. "I just have a feeling."

"I really think you need to come in now."

"Can't do it," he says.

"Can you tell me why?"

"I just—I want to go home. I've lived with this a long time, and I think it's going to be okay, tonight."

I sigh. Why does he have to do this?

"I would have to say that's against our advice."

"Emily—Dr. Emily—I understand that. And I appreciate your concern. But it's my life, and my illness, and I'm going home."

His eyes are calm and clear, looking into mine, and I realize that further talk is not going to get me anywhere. I nod slowly. "I'm sorry. I think you should stay. But if you're set on leaving, I'll get you papers to sign. . . ."

He nods.

When my shift is over, I go home to bed, falling into sleep like a starved person falling on a plate of food. I wake seven hours later, my head still full of uneasy ER dreams, feeling only partly refreshed.

There are still a few hours left before I'm supposed to be at work. I dress and wander up to Broadway, the busy shopping street near my apartment. It's rained during the day while I slept, but the sun is out now, and the air is wet and fresh.

Before this month started, knowing it would be among the busiest of these busy three years, I prepared. Strange preparations the logic of which I cannot entirely explain. I filled my freezer with little canisters of homemade soup, and my fruit basket with sweet potatoes—the only thing I could think of that wouldn't spoil. I paid my bills, organized two years' worth of papers, sent out a month's worth of early birthday cards. I went to the doctor and the dentist, got my hair cut, changed my car's oil. I scoured my apartment from floor to ceiling.

As a result, in my hours away from work, I find that I have very little of life's ordinary business to do. It's strange not to have errands. I wander down Broadway past the places I usually go, realizing I have no need for them. I can't even think of anything to buy. Books, but I have no time to read them; music when I want only silence; movies when I am so overloaded with real drama that I couldn't stand a Hollywood reenactment. Broadway, with its throngs of normal people and normal things, has nothing to offer me in one sense and is everything I need in another.

I breathe in deeply the smell of coffee from the espresso place on the corner. There is an almost hallucinatory state I fall into when I am overworked and overtired. Every emotion, every sensation seems amplified. After my nights in the ER, in particular, everything outside seems strangely bright and polished. At the smell of the coffee, my head floods with unexpected memories. Paris, Florence, the cup of Turkish coffee I drank one early morning waiting for a bus from Sofia, Bulgaria, up to a monastery in the mountains. The next breath smells more of mist than coffee, and suddenly I am thinking of New Zealand, of the incredible green hills after a rain.

Still awash in a parade of images and memories, I walk by a policeman pulling a man out of a car. I find myself glancing to see if I know either of them. Is that one of the cops I've seen in the ER? Is the guy he's picking up one of our regulars?

I realize that I'm on edge, waiting for a voice to say "Dr. Emily!" As it has sometimes, when I've been walking down Broadway in the afternoon—a couple of off-duty nurses once, patients other times. But today it doesn't happen.

I walk past the flower shop, noticing with great vividness and clarity the smells, the color and shape of each petal. The roses with their whorls of velvet color, the hyacinths with each bell shaped and ordered in its place. Was anything ever such a dark green or pale pink, so deep a blue or pale an apricot?

Walking farther down the street, I find myself enjoying each face as it passes, studying them in snapshots, imagining sketches. I remember back to my drawing days, studying lines, the angle of a jaw, a neck, the shape of a nose. Will I ever draw again? I wonder.

I pass a shop window full of slinky, sexy little dresses. In another incarnation of my life, I might have bought these to wear salsa dancing into the wee hours of the morning. Sometimes I long for an irresponsible life.

I pick up a copy of the local paper, which I will study later like an anthropologist reading documents from another culture. I peek into the Gap to see what normal clothes look like these days. I've only been in the ER for a few weeks, but it feels like years, like the whole outside world might have changed without my knowing it.

I stop at Taco Bell. I've been living on frozen soup and sweet potatoes, at home and reheated at the hospital. Though I'm not really hungry, I decide that a taco would be good for me. There's a young man—twentyish, strong-looking—taking orders with prideful efficiency. "You're next in line—make it snappy, come on, come on!" I tell him I want a soft taco and a small Sprite, and he rings up my order with flourish. "One seventy-three! Okay, who's next? . . ."

Meanwhile five people in front of me are waiting for their orders. In the back is a tiny, heavyset woman, plodding along, making up order after order, one piece at a time, all alone. I look at her—her shuffling gait, the slightly odd alignment of her face—and know there's something wrong with her. Some developmental disability or neurologic disease.

He doesn't help her. He sits there at the front counter waiting for more orders, while customers pile up waiting for their food, and she stands there, slowly and miserably attempting to assemble burritos.

I find myself furious, as if my tolerance for injustice had been used up in my nights in the ER—nights of senseless pain and death and horror—and I have none left for the outside. I have a moment of blinding hatred in which I could almost reach across the counter and slam the boy's head into the cold hard metal, punish him for being such a dolt, for being so pleased with himself for the pointless speed of his orders while this poor deformed woman in the back struggles away at her hopeless task.

I bite into my taco, which is dry and plain, and realize I should have spent the extra twenty cents to get tomatoes. How can they charge you extra for tomatoes on a taco? And on the other hand, how could I skip them over a lousy twenty cents. . . .

I remember an incident the night before in the cafeteria. I'd run down to grab a roll to go with my reheated soup and was delayed because of a fuss in the line in front of me. A middle-aged woman was there with her child, about eight. They each had a hot dog and a drink, and the little girl had a Dove bar, carried carefully by the edge. They got to the front of the line and didn't have enough money to pay for it.

The mother said she'd take the hot dog back and the cashier said no, she couldn't do that, there was already ketchup on it. In the end it was the Dove bar—the one thing still in packaging—that was put back, the little girl's face crumpling as she was forced to hand it over.

Through it all I had the sickening sense that this had happened before, that it wasn't an accident that there wasn't enough money, that it was all some kind of awful game or gamble—though whether the goal was to make the cashier pass them through, or elicit a contribution from the audience, or whether it was somehow aimed at teaching the girl some kind of lesson, I couldn't say. The whole incident was sinister and awful.

And I can't figure out why I didn't just pay for the little girl's Dove bar. What could have been simpler? It would have been worth ten times its cost to have seen the child smile, to be spared the sight of her fallen face as she relinquished the ice cream. It wasn't that I couldn't or wouldn't spare the money. It just didn't occur to me to offer, not until later, not until now. What was I thinking, I wonder? But I wasn't thinking. I was so tired, standing in line with no more power to act inside me than a video camera recording the scene. I have a sudden terrible knowledge that I will regret that moment for my entire life, that I will carry with me always the child's pain and the fact that I could so easily have prevented it. Two dollars. Not reaching out with two dollars will buy me a place in hell.

Twenty cents for tomatoes and two dollars for a little girl's happiness—how can I be trusted with people's lives when I can't correctly judge such simple things as these?

HEADING HOME, I get caught up in the smell of shrubs and flowers after the rain. I pass through a sweet smell, then a spicy one, so perfect, so complete. It's such a strange state, this hypersensitivity of fatigue; in a funny way I enjoy it, long for it when it's gone.

It's almost a relief to be back in the ER. I get caught up quickly in the whirl of it, three people with chest pain, one with pneumonia, one with fever and pain on urination, probably an infection.

Setting the urine sample down on the back counter, my eyes catch on a discarded label sitting next to it. The name catches my attention: the seizure guy, the guy from last night. The date on the sticker is today.

It has to be him. It's not a common name. Anxiety grips me—tell me something terrible didn't happen, that he's okay, that I shouldn't have tried harder to . . .

"Peter Maartin. Was he here again today?" I ask the secretary at the desk.

"Who?"

"Maartin. Peter Maartin." I hand her the sticker.

She peers at it. My heart pounds.

"Oh, yeah," she says. "He went up to Neuro."

"Was he okay?"

"He was a direct admit. Dr. Olson. She saw him in clinic and wanted to bring him in, but she decided to send him through here for some labs." She rolls her eyes. Damn clinic docs who don't know how to admit someone without using up the ER's time, her expression says.

Then she looks up. "That's right—I remember now. He asked after you. Dr. Emily. I said you were on nights."

She gives me a curious look. I shrug. "He was here last night. I wanted to admit him but he wouldn't come in. I'm just glad he's okay."

She nods. "Seemed fine."

I savor my sense of relief for a few seconds, then struggle with another dilemma. I want to go up to the floor and check on him. It occurs to me that maybe I shouldn't go up, maybe there would be something strange or wrong or irregular about that. Then I think: I've gone to see lots of other ER patients who were admitted. Why should this guy be different, just because he made me smile?

"Hi," he says with a bright smile, as I walk in.

"I saw you came in."

"Yep."

"So you saw Dr. Olson in clinic," I say.

"She said the same thing you said. Not that I didn't trust you—"

"I know," I say.

"I wasn't ready to come in yesterday. I . . . I can't explain."

"I understand," I say. "It's okay. You're all right, that's the important thing."

There's a pause. He glances at me, his expression uncertain. It's so quiet up here, so calm, and suddenly I realize I'm scared, or at least a little nervous. The bustle and craziness of the ER provided more of a shield than I'd realized. I feel less comfortable now, more vulnerable. Here it's almost—private.

"So how old *are* you?" he asks suddenly.

I wonder for an instant if it's okay to answer this. It's not like it's a tremendously personal question. I've told lots of patients how old I am. It's not a big deal, just a little friendly gesture.

But some inner voice tells me no. That while I wouldn't be crossing any lines, it's better not to put myself in a position of having to decide where to draw them. Better to stop before starting.

So I just smile and shake my head. Then I say, "I've got to get back down to the ER. I just wanted to make sure you were okay."

And he nods and says, "Thanks . . ." His smile seems real.

I shake his hand and turn to go. Just as I'm slipping out his doorway, he murmurs thoughtfully, almost wonderingly: "That time you almost told me. . . ."

And it's true. I almost did.

I walk down the hallway, shaking my head, still confused by this whole business, but beginning to understand that this, too, will be part of my life, something to learn to accept and live with. It occurs to me that I will always be grateful to Peter Maartin, if nothing else, for saving me from marrying Kevin, or anyone like Kevin. I'll hold out for chemistry. It's got to happen with someone else eventually. Someone who's not a patient, please, next time.

I wrap my stethoscope around my neck and step back into the ER, which suddenly seems like a very simple and predictable world.

34. Mania

I heard her—everyone in the ER heard her—before seeing her. She was audible the moment the wide front doors swung open to let her pass.

"I am under eighteen years old. You cannot do anything to me without my parents being present. I do not want to be here. I am not coming in here. You do not have a right to bring me here. I want to leave. I want to go home. I want to talk to my lawyer."

She's a tiny thing, I realize, looking up as she walks by. Not much above five feet, with a wiry, compact frame, braided head held high. Her hands are tied behind her back. She is flanked by two policemen, two hospital guards, and another two men in an unfamiliar uniform. The little procession files by, headed toward the seclusion room at the end of the hall. I don't hear anything except her voice, continuing its monologue, until they reach the room. Then I hear screaming and a scuffle, and then silence as they close the soundproof door.

I don't want any piece of that, I think to myself ungenerously.

Whatever that situation is, somebody else can damn well deal with it. Then the attending hands me her chart. Some of the ER attendings with whom I work make a principle of taking cases like this—messy things, half psych and half legal, not a lot of medicine involved. But this guy hands off anything that seems like trouble.

I accept the chart, forcing a smile. "Medical clearance for juvenile detention," it notes, not offering me any further details. I look for her age: thirteen.

I go in to talk to her, but they're drawing her blood. This translates into six people holding her down, a towel wrapped around her head to keep her from biting or bashing into anything, while two people hold her arm trying to get it still enough for a nurse to get a needle into. I can't watch. I leave her chart on my pile and start working up another patient.

I wait until the nurse has emerged, victorious, with two vials of blood before braving that end of the hallway again. Two guards are flanking the door; those unfamiliar uniforms must be from juvenile detention. I peer into the little window on her door. She's stretched on the bed, one arm tied above her head, the other to her side, her legs at the foot of the bed. She is quite still except for her mouth, which is moving steadily. I can faintly hear her voice though the soundproofing.

"She's been going like that since three this afternoon," says one of the guards.

"Be careful," adds the other as I reach for the doorknob. "She spits."

With a deep breath, I open the door. Her voice continues, unchanged in pitch or speed by my entrance.

"I am not crazy. I am not a criminal. I have not done anything wrong. You do not have the right to do anything to me. I do not give you permission to touch me. I do not give you permission to examine me. I want to be in another room right now. I want the restraints taken off of me right now. I want to be in a room with a television and a phone. I want to make some phone calls."

She takes a breath. "I want a restraining order. I want those people to stop following me. Those people do not have any right to be following me. I have not done anything wrong. You can ask my probation officer. I don't want to be at this hospital I don't like this hospital I have my own doctor I have my own hospital I have a right to be seen by my own doctor even if it is an emergency.

"I had an exam last week there's nothing wrong with me I am not sick I am not crazy I do not want to be examined, I want you to take the restraints off me right now I want to be placed in another room right now I want to leave I want to go home I want a glass of juice, I want a phone I want a television I want something to eat I want you to go away."

I wait to see if she'll stop on her own. She doesn't. "Look," I say finally. "Can I talk to you for just a minute?"

"No you can't talk to me. I'm doing the talking here. I don't want to hear anything you have to say. You people have assaulted me. I want to be let out of here. I want to go home."

"I'm sorry," I say. "I just need to talk to you for a sec."

She pauses just long enough to shoot me a suspicious frown. "You're trying to be the nice guy. I don't want to talk to you. You're just trying to trick information out of me. I am not crazy. I am not a criminal. I do not sell drugs anymore. My past is behind me. You cannot do anything to me."

"I'm not involved in any of that, do you understand? I don't care about your past. I don't know what happened at the juvenile center. I'm just here to make sure there isn't something medically wrong with you."

"The only thing that's wrong with me is that people have been hassling me all day and I'm sick of it." She stops at last, with emphasis on the last phrase.

I have to hide a smile. "I'm sorry about that," I say. "And I'm sorry to be part of hassling you some more. But I have to ask you a couple of questions."

She frowns, but she stays quiet.

"What's the date?"

"You guys keep asking me that."

"I know. I'm sorry. But I have to ask you again."

"I'm not going to tell you."

"Fine." I sigh.

"It's the ninth. Of May."

"Thank you," I say.

"Nineteen ninety mother-fucking eight!"

The interview goes on in similar fashion. I gather that she'd been down at the juvenile detention center this morning, checking in as ordered with her probation officer. She'd felt some people there were following her, and she had gotten upset. She won't specify what happened after that to land her here. The guards will tell me later she attacked someone. She says she's taken some marijuana today but nothing else, a fact which will be confirmed by her tox screens.

After I've gotten all the information she's willing or able to give me, I say I need to do a quick exam.

She screams as I reach toward her. "Don't touch me!"

I step back. "This is a stethoscope." I hold it out to her. "I need to listen to your heart and your lungs, okay?"

Reluctantly she lets me listen.

"Now I'm going to feel your belly, and check your lymph nodes."

She doesn't answer, but she doesn't scream as I reach toward her.

The neuro exam is harder, between the fact that she's tied to the bed, and that she won't cooperate with anything I ask. I do what I can, then turn to leave.

"I'm going to go check on your lab results, and then I'll be back, okay?"

She jerks into sudden animation. "Don't give them any of my blood. Don't give them anything. They already have my fingerprints, I don't want them having any of my blood."

"Your blood will be used for some basic medical tests," I say. "To see if you're sick. That's all."

"I'm not sick," she says. "I'm not crazy."

I know it's pointless, but I try to explain. "Some people who act the way you're acting have something wrong in their head. An infection. Even a tumor. And they can act like this, and not even know that that's why it is. And until I can say for sure that there isn't anything like that going on, I can't let you leave."

"There's nothing wrong in my head," she insists.

"I appreciate that you think that," I say. "But I have to prove it before I can let you go."

I step toward the door.

"I want to sit up!" she screams. "I want some juice."

"I'll get you some juice," I say wearily. "And I'll try to get someone to help you sit up."

I walk back past her guards carrying a cup of juice.

"Careful. The other times people have taken juice in there she just spits it all over the place."

"Well, I'm going to try," I say. I'm not sure if I'm more exasperated at her or at him.

She drinks the juice down quietly.

"I want to sit up," she says after she finishes.

"I'm working on that," I say. "We will if we can."

"I'm not sick. I'm not crazy!" she screams after me as I shut the door.

"Is there any reason we can't let her sit up?" I say quietly to the guard.

"She has to have one arm restrained over her head."

I frown.

"If she doesn't, she can move enough to bash her head against the wall, which is what she was doing earlier."

"*Fuck,*" I murmur to myself.

"How's your crazy kid in there?" my attending asks cheerfully.

I sigh. "I don't know," I say. "Such a messy situation. Poor kid."

"She's psychotic," he says.

What do you know? I want to ask. You wouldn't even go in there.

"She's manic. I don't know if I'd say psychotic. She has pressured speech, sure, and a little paranoid ideation, although given everything I'm not sure how dissociated from reality that really is. I mean, she says the people from the youth center are following her and not leaving her alone. And they are following her and not leaving her alone, aren't they?"

He gives me a look that says I'm starting to sound crazy, myself.

I START CALLING consults. Psych sees her, says that she's probably manic, that it's unlikely to be caused by the marijuana. Without any indication that she's going to kill herself or someone else, they can't do much. They make her a follow-up appointment in two weeks. Great, I think. That helps.

The exhausted and overworked social worker says that she's a pain in the ass, and she should go back to the pediatric jail.

God, I think to myself, I hate this. More than any other piece of my work, I hate this.

My own anger at the situation momentarily overwhelms me. I realize that I'm going to have to get a grip on my own emotions before I can attempt to handle hers. I have to do lots of things in my job that I don't like; why does this one get to me so particularly?

I tick the reasons off on my fingers. I hate forcing anyone into anything. One of the reasons I chose internal medicine over pediatrics or psychiatry was that the overwhelming majority of my patients, unlike theirs, are competent to consent or refuse. You can try to talk people into things, but ultimately if they say no, you walk away. I understand that there are situations like this one when those rights have to be overridden—emergencies, times when someone's mental competence is in question—but I still hate being part of it. I hate treating her as if she was violent or self-destructive when I haven't seen her be either of those things, when I wasn't around in the original situation to see what really happened.

Most of all, I hate the ambiguous position of responsibility for her I am placed in. I know that she needs help—psychiatric, or social, or very likely both. She probably doesn't need medical help. She's been put under my auspices for the purpose of ruling out medical illness, but we all know that the chances of my finding anything are very small. The things that make adolescents act crazy are drugs, mental illness, and social or behavioral problems, not tumors and infections. She's been placed in my care for problems she almost certainly doesn't have, while I don't have the skills or authority to deal with the problems she does have. Feeling responsible for someone who desperately needs help, but not being able to give it to them, is hardly a formula for job satisfaction.

I pull up her labs on the computer. Her white blood count is significantly elevated. Probably just a stress response from all the excitement, but . . .

The attending is talking to the social worker as I walk up to him. "Ms. Lewis is just waiting for her labs, and then she'll be cleared to go wherever she's going."

"Ms. Lewis has a white count of seventeen," I say quietly.

He turns with a pained expression and says what I'm thinking: "So we need to CT and LP her."

I nod. We? I want to say. What do you have to do with it?

"Yes."

"She'll need to be sedated."

"Yes."

I don't want to sedate her. The last thing I want is to tie her down, drug her, scan her head, and stick a needle in her back for spinal fluid, which is what I'm about to do.

I have no choice, though. The options have closed in on both of us. What if I didn't do it and she came back the next day with some florid nervous system infection, unconscious or even dead, or with permanent brain damage? What if she did turn out to have a burst blood vessel or a tumor and she went back to detention and died? It's very unlikely, but there's no way that I can run that risk.

As I walk down the hallway toward her room, I think about William Carlos Williams's famous story of the girl with diphtheria. I too am about to use force to overcome a child, though in a very different setting. I have the luxury of distancing myself: I don't have to be the one to hold her down, to conquer her. I just say to the nurse: "Ms. Lewis needs an IV. And Valium in five-milligram increments as needed to calm her down for a CT scan and an LP."

The nurse nods slowly. "Okay." I hear both the weariness and the resignation in her voice.

"I'm sorry," I say.

"Not your fault."

Then I get to walk away and not watch what happens next, not watch them hold her down, the whole process of the blood draw again, only worse, because they have to get an IV to stay in, this time. Instead, I go evaluate a couple of drunks and a woman with belly pain. Things I feel more or less equipped to handle.

By the time I return, the IV is in, the Valium given. Now that she's been massively sedated, they've taken off the restraints and moved her out of the seclusion room.

But she's still talking, a little more slowly and a lot more quietly, but still nonstop. It's as if the Valium just turned down her volume knob. She's gone from a 10 to a 1, but it's the same record.

"What have you done to me you're giving me stuff and it's making me feel weird and maybe I'm having a bad reaction and I don't want you to give me any more of that stuff and I want to be left alone and I want to get out of here. . . ." She tosses on the bed.

"Give her another five milligrams," I say.

THE CT SCAN isn't quite normal.

"It's almost normal," the radiologist says, peering at it. "But there's one area here that's a little funny, and I can't say for sure. If you're worried, we should probably get a contrast CT to follow up, just to be safe."

" 'Probably?' " I ask. She knows I need a yes or no.

"She needs the contrast scan," she says.

The guards are restless. "Do you know when you'll be done, Doc?" one asks, glancing at his watch.

I shake my head. "It's really hard to say. Depends on the results of the scan, and so on."

"You look tired, Doc," he says, smiling gently at me.

He looks like a nice man. This is crazy, I think to myself. How did she, and he, and I all get into this crazy situation? She's an adolescent and she's having a manic break and what she needs is to be admitted to some nice psych ward and kept safe and started on some medication. Or maybe she's just wildly worked up and acting out and what she needs is to go home and go to bed. But instead, we're going to run her through our medical mill, poke and prod and drug and needle her, declare that she doesn't have any of the organic causes of mania that would be vanishingly rare in a healthy young kid anyway—and then she's going to jail.

THE CONTRAST CT—after another round of Valium and another hour or two of waiting for the scan to be done and read—is normal. I go in to do her lumbar puncture.

She's lying on the bed, silent for the first time that I've seen her, breathing easily. She looks so young, now that she's asleep. Her face has softened into childish lines, her braided hair reminds me of the girls I knew in grade school. She's only a baby. She looks as young as the brain-dead twelve-year-old I once watched an organ harvest on. Jesus, why did I come up with that image?

The nurse holds her in a loose curl while I prep her for the tap. She moans softly, tosses. As I slide the lidocaine needle into her back she jerks and cries out—how much Valium have we poured into this tiny little body, I wonder, and she's still not asleep.

"More Valium," I say.

After the tap, as I cover the needle site with a small bandage, I wonder what she'll think in the morning. She'll wake up with a headache and a band-aid in the small of her back, probably some vague memories of being drugged and stuck with needles and run through giant, whirring machines. God only knows what she'll conclude from all of that. Is it too naive to hope she'll recall only a blur? Or will the experiences of this night be enough to convince her forever that there are vastly powerful evil forces allied against her?

The spinal fluid results show just a few too many white blood cells. Not enough to make me really think it's meningitis, but too many to let me declare her normal and send her home. That is, send her to jail, or whatever is in store for her.

Meanwhile, she's sound asleep, snoring quietly on her stretcher. "Has she woken up at all?" I ask her nurse, a little anxiously. I hope we didn't give her too much Valium, after all that.

"Not really," the nurse says. "She tosses and turns a little." She looks at the girl protectively. "She must be so worn out. She'd been going like that nonstop all day. I'd think she'd sleep a long time."

I look at my watch; it's 3:30 A.M. I suppose it would be normal for her to be sleeping soundly even without the Valium, even if she hadn't had a day like this one. I could use some sleep, myself. I've been here for fourteen hours, I have to be back in ten. I'm not thinking straight.

I call the Neurology team to admit her. It won't change much. They'll watch her for a day, repeat the lab tests and maybe the spinal tap, then send her back to juvenile detention. But at least I know she'll be watched tonight and have clearer heads than mine looking after her.

Driving home through the dark streets, I struggle with a lingering, painful dissatisfaction. I can't help feeling that somehow I could have, should have, managed all this differently. I review each step and can't find any medical mistakes, can't even find a point at which I had the choice to do things some other way. Yet somehow a child in terrible distress came to us, and I'm afraid that we left her even more brutalized than when she came. I see her again, walking in through the front door, her head held high, flanked by her hostile entourage; crazy, maybe, but proud and defiant also, in a way I have to admire. What have I done to her?

Before I fall asleep I take *The Doctor Stories* off my shelf, trying to remember how Williams's story ends. His child is clawing and furious in her defeat. Mine, thanks to technology, is sleeping, an artificial, drug-induced peace. If this is a victory, it is one in which I take little comfort.

35. Drunk Alley

They're here every night, some old, some young, some new, some only too familiar. The first ones come around 6:00 P.M., and more drift in throughout the night, a few staggering in of their own accord, most brought by ambulance or the police. Anyone found out there too drunk to walk or talk comes on in to the ER.

They have their own space, not a glamorous one. They lie on stretchers lining a back hallway. Drunk Alley, it's called. We check them quickly, make sure there's nothing more serious going on than alcohol, draw a blood alcohol level, give them a shot of thiamine, and let them sleep it off. Early in the morning, around five-thirty, we go down the line, wake them all up, send them on their way.

It's usually pretty quiet in Drunk Alley—most of the patients are passed out, a few mumble quietly to themselves—but it can get raucous. There's a famous anecdote in my program about someone who's now a doc at the university hospital, a quiet, sweet woman, full of smiles. When she was a resident in the ER, she was walking down Drunk Alley at the end of a shift and someone yelled at her, "Hey, bitch!"—a not uncommon epithet in that part of the ER. She spun on him, and snapped, "That's *Doctor* Bitch to you!"

But there's another side to it, a stranger side. A lot of these guys are regulars here. They come in every few weeks, or every week, some almost every night. By the end of my first week, I know a lot of the guys in Drunk Alley; by the end of the month, I know most of them. The nurses who work here know them all. They know their stories, things about them that you would never expect. Despite occasional sparring on both sides—a new resident with a bad attitude toward these dirty and needy and down-and-out patients, a patient getting violent in the throes of intoxication or withdrawal—the relationship overall between the ER staff and the alcoholics is a remarkably cordial one. I sense affection on both sides. The ER serves as a kind of strange, dysfunctional home and family to some of these unfortunate people. Here at least they can find warmth and a bed and a little to eat; here there are familiar people who are kind and who will not turn them away.

I'm signing one man out one morning, a particularly frequent offender. He's here practically every night. I wake him up, and he shuffles to his feet and stretches. "Where's my knife?" he asks sleepily.

I open my mouth to say, "We don't hand out weapons in the ER, sir," but an answer comes from behind me. "It's right here, with your other things," the nurse says quietly. "Don't worry."

She hands him his bag and he nods and scuffles away. I turn to her. "His *knife*?"

"He carves," she says.

My face must betray my incredulity. How could this man carve and not cut his fingers off? He's here every night, he'll be back here in twelve hours smashed out of his mind. He probably starts drinking on our doorstep.

"He's very good," the nurse says, wearily. "He did one of the big statues on the riverfront downtown. You should ask him to let you look at some of his stuff sometime—it's beautiful, very intricate. Ask him in the morning, of course, not at night. He's in a better mood."

She smiles and walks away, leaving my jaw still hanging.

Pete is another one I know, another one we all know. I see his name on the board and put my initials next to it. "Well known within this system," I'll write in his note.

"How ya doing tonight, Pete?" I ask, putting my stethoscope to his chest.

"Not so good," he murmurs, slurring thickly.

"How come?" I ask.

"Fell," he says.

He points to his face, and I see that he's bleeding. Mixed with all the dirt on his face, there is blood as well. I trace the bleeding to a jagged gash over one eyebrow.

"Bumped myself," he murmurs sadly.

I explore the cut. It's fairly deep, and more than an inch long. "We'll have to have the surgeons have a look at that," I say. He nods. He's been through this before.

The surgeons are all tied up in the trauma rooms with a couple of gunshot wounds that just came in. They won't have time tonight for head bumps. It occurs to me that, though the surgeons usually handle lacerations here, I'm more than capable of sewing up a cut like this.

"Change of plan," I say, coming back. "I'm going to fix that up for you."

I gather suture, drapes, saline rinse, antiseptic, and a syringe. I clean him up carefully, drape his head, and begin a row of careful stitches.

I'm interrupted by a voice from further down the alley.

"Hey, *Doc!*" one of the other patients shouts.

I look up. He's another one I'm looking after. "Sir . . . I'm a little busy right now, okay?"

"Okay," he says. "But—"

"I'll be with you just as soon as I'm done with this."

"Okay," he says again, his voice barely below a yell, "but Doc—"

I glare at him, and return to my work.

"Could you just tell Pete I said hi?"

I'm trying to make sense of this statement—*tell who what?*—when I'm distracted by a sudden motion under my hands. The head I'm sewing on is moving, rising—Christ, he's sitting up!

"That voice!" he shouts. "I know that voice!"

I shove him rather indelicately back down onto the bed. "Please, *sit down!*"

He lies back, but continues: "What is that voice?!"

The man down the hall calls back, "Pete! Pete! It's me, George!"

"George?"

"Pete!"

"George!"

"Pete!"

"Could you please hold still?" I interject.

"Sure, sure," he mumbles. "Hey, George," he adds at a yell, "what the hell have you been up to?"

"Oh, this and that," answers George, managing somehow to mumble and yell at the same time. "I tried to come by your house the other day. What's her name, that woman, that . . ."

"My wife," supplies Pete.

"Your wife. She said you were at rehab."

"I don't think he's in rehab anymore," I murmur under my breath. What was his alcohol level? Four hundred something?

"Man," Pete says, "it's been a long time. How long's it been, George?"

"Couple months, I think," says George. "Remember back a couple months ago, we were in detox together?"

Pete starts laughing, his head shaking under my hands as I tie his sutures. "Man, that was the best . . ."

"This is all very touching," I interject, "but could you hold still for just one more minute?"

I finish sewing Pete's forehead, and they both sleep for a few hours. I'm working on paperwork when one of the nurses calls to me, "A couple of guys in the back want to talk to you. They have a question."

I go back. "Um, Doc . . ." Pete gives me a big, uncertain smile.

"Yes?"

George fills in for him. "Hey, you know, we were just wondering. . . . Well, whenever you guys decide it's okay for us to go . . . do you think you could let us out together?"

"Please?" adds Pete.

I look from the one to the other. "You want me . . . to let you go . . . together . . . so that you can go out . . . and have . . ." I give them each one last glance before finishing the sentence. "A drink."

"Oh, no, Doc," Pete asserts.

"Of course not," says George.

"We wouldn't."

"No," I say. "Of course you wouldn't."

"Please, Doc?"

I groan. What am I supposed to do? I've offered them both detox or rehab and they've both refused. Ah, what the hell . . . I sign them out together. At least they won't be drinking alone.

As I finish Pete's note it occurs to me that I didn't tell him to come back in a few days to have his stitches out. I feel a pang of guilt, then realize that I needn't worry. He'll be back, probably more than once, before the stitches are mature. He's never gone for long.

36. Counting

The transition from the second year of residency to the third is not a dramatic one. The rotations are a little different: more ICU time, less medical wards, more electives. Everyone around you is going through big changes. The residents above you are leaving to start fellowship or practice. Last year's interns are blossoming into R2's, and a new set of interns are coming—the generation who were third-year students during your internship. Your last July.

But for you, it's not a big change, just another milestone to check off. Two years down, one to go.

The medical profession puts labels on people who count too much. We call them obsessive-compulsive: people who count the red jellybeans in the bag or the number of steps on the walk to work. But every medical resident I know counts obsessively.

It began, for me, with months. I counted the number of months I had in internship, and how many of those were call months. (Thirteen and three, respectively. The internship "months" are actually four-week blocks, coming out to thirteen in a year instead of twelve. A cruel trick, as far as we were concerned.) I checked them off as they went by. "I am two weeks and three days into my seventh month of internship." Then there were call nights to be counted: how many left in the month, the year. With three months remaining I expanded the count to hours on call.

There were other things to count. Shifts in the ER, holidays on call, days till the next day off. The number of patients I was taking care of at a given time, how many of those would be leaving by the next call night, how many would stay. How many hours until I could expect to leave the hospital. How many notes to be written each day, how many labs to be checked, how many phone calls needing to be made. My fellow residents and I made endless to-do lists with little check boxes, and we counted as we checked the boxes off. If there were things I had done that weren't on the list, I would add them, just to improve the ratio.

So the chance to mark off another year, the second of three, was no small thing. Two-thirds done! I was tired by then, and drifting on the edges of depression. One more year. Anyone can do anything for a year.

It would strike me later that I remembered less from my second and third years than from internship. Partly this was because things were less new, so not every memory had the vividness of novelty. Partly it was because I had less direct patient contact. Since I supervised more and talked to patients less, they didn't always imprint as deeply on my consciousness. Sometimes, also, I succumbed to burnout, let myself think of my patients as check boxes instead of people with stories. Luckily it was never long before they pulled me back to reality again.

After I finished residency, counting was one of the hardest things to unlearn. It took an existential shift to cease envisioning my life in terms of blocks to be checked off, days to be gotten through. Ironically, residency taught me to see life as a precious and tenuous thing, one that could be snatched from anyone at any moment. Yet it put me in the habit of treating my own life like an obstacle course, a series of unpleasant tasks to be raced through as quickly as possible, as if it was the end and not the process that was important.

People have asked, at the time and since, whether I liked residency. The question baffles me as much now as it did then. Am I glad I did it? Yes. I never learned as much or grew as much in any three years, and never will. Would I do it again? No. I can't conceive of mustering that kind of energy again. Once in a lifetime was enough. Was it pleasant? No, on the whole, though moments were. It was satisfying, sometimes fun, but never easy.

Was it horrible? No. Still, by the third year I was counting hours, and at the end I counted minutes.

37. Abscess

She's twenty-one, but she looks about twelve. Beautiful, with big dark eyes and long glossy hair, thin, fragile-looking. And obviously terrified.

She's been shooting heroin for only three months, and she already has an abscess—bad luck, probably, or maybe bad procedure. Maybe the abscess is even good luck, since it's scared her and brought her in here. Her slender, bony forearm is swollen to almost double its normal circumference, and there's a round, hard spot about two centimeters across where you can feel the collection of pus under her skin.

She stares wide-eyed while I prep the area with sterilizing solution, drape it with sterile towels. "You're sure it won't hurt?" she asks anxiously.

I'm always fascinated by the low tolerance that heroin addicts have for pain, their frequent terrible fear of needles. "The numbing medication will sting, like it does at the dentist. Then you won't feel anything but pressure."

She chats nervously as I prepare the lidocaine. "I'm not supposed to get these things," she says. "I just started using, and I never skin-pop—I have great veins," she adds proudly.

I wonder who taught her to be proud of this, and whether they also told her that this habit would replace them with scarred track marks soon enough. "You do now," I say, a little severely. "You won't for very long if you don't get some help."

She hangs her head.

She whimpers as I inject the lidocaine and watches with a kind of curious detachment as I cut into her arm and the pus gushes out. She doesn't say anything until I have packed the wound and told her how to care for it. She repeats the instructions back to me dully.

As I am laying a final gauze over the wound and taping it, she pipes up suddenly: "How big will the bandage be?"

"About like this." I measure with my fingers.

"That's too big," she says.

"What do you mean?"

"My mother can't see it," she says matter-of-factly. "I live at home."

I fight the urge to say, why the hell hasn't your mother noticed what's going on already?

Instead I say, "Maybe this is the time to talk to her about all this."

She shakes her head. "I'll just wear long sleeves."

I urge her to see our social worker about drug treatment and rehab, but she shakes her head. "I have to get home, I'm late," she says gaily. "Maybe I'll come back another time."

I suspect you will, I think to myself as she slips away.

38. Blackberries

I was spending a month on an oncology elective. One day we saw a young woman in her thirties who had a history of cervical cancer, three years before. She'd just discovered a new lump in her groin.

I talked to her first, before the attending came in. She's beautiful, slender, with long dark hair and dark eyes. You could see tension running through her every movement, every gesture. She'd found the lump a week before. It was hard but not painful. Yesterday she thought she could feel a second one.

"So you're a Medicine R-Three?" she asked, while we waited for the attending.

It was a question a medical professional would ask, so after I nodded I asked, "What do you do?"

"I'm an anesthesiologist."

"Excellent. Where?"

She names a local hospital.

"Do you like it there?"

"Mostly. There's politics, of course, and all that crap. But it's a good field. It's stressful, but we get paid well and have a decent life."

She pauses on "life," and looks stricken. Knowledge can be a terrible thing. She knows what I know: that her lumps are almost certainly metastases, a recurrence of the cancer.

The attending comes in and she smiles, a frightened but trusting smile. He takes her hand reassuringly. He hears the story, feels her lumps and nods. "Well, we better get a CT to see what's going on there. We'll see you back next week to go over the results."

He asks her about work and they have a brief talk about the hospital. I notice how she seems less frightened, less fragile as she moves into the role of a professional talking to a colleague rather than a patient talking to a doctor.

ONCOLOGY BOTH DRAWS and repels me. The patients are wonderful, the science of fighting tumors is wonderful. For the first week of every oncology rotation I think I should subspecialize in it. By the second week I start to get tired, and by the third I have trouble getting out of bed in the morning. General medicine has enough of a mix of the tragic and the mundane to keep me going, but oncology does not.

THE NEXT WEEK she's back, and I go into her room while the attending goes to get the CT from radiology.

"I saw you the other day. At the park," she says.

I am confused. "What?"

"You were—I'm sure it was you—at Magnussen Park. You know, Magnussen Park."

Was I?

"Yes," I remember suddenly. "Yes, I was."

"You were wearing white shorts. And driving a little green—a green—"

There's an edge of desperation in her voice. "A green Honda," I say. "Yes. And white shorts, I remember. I—I was picking blackberries."

"I was sure it was you!" she says. "I knew it. Even though I only saw you from behind."

"I was there," I say. "I didn't see you," I add apologetically.

"That's okay. But I knew you were there."

THE ATTENDING WALKS in with the CT. "Do you want to look at it, or do you want me to just talk it through?"

"Just tell me."

He nods. "The nodes in your groin aren't alone. There's diffuse involvement in the pelvis as well as the retroperitoneum."

She gives a brisk, fierce nod. I can see that she was prepared for this, and has decided not to cry. "What are we doing to do?"

"Radiation will slow it down," he says carefully.

"You're telling me I'm going to die of this."

There's a long pause. Finally he says simply, "Yes."

A small eternity passes in silence.

He adds, "Realistically, we knew all along there was a good possibility that this would happen."

She starts to cry.

"I don't want to drown in my own secretions—I don't want to die like that. I don't want to die not being able to breathe—"

"That's not going to happen. I promise you, that's not going to happen."

"I don't want to die in terrible pain—"

Her voice is panicked now, veering toward hysteria. "I don't want bedsores. I've seen people with bedsores. I don't want to be like that—"

He takes her hand and quiets her like a child. "Shh, shhhh . . . It isn't time to think like that. Right now it's time to fight. And when later comes, we'll deal with all those things. You know we will. Don't worry."

"What happens when I get malnourished? Will you give me intravenous nutrition? A feeding tube?"

"Shh! We'll do whatever you want and need. We don't know how far off that is. Concentrate on now."

"Should I keep working?"

He smiles ruefully.

"I know you're going to tell me you can't answer that. But I can't seem to answer it for myself. I just can't."

"You'll figure it out," he says. "Just give it time."

"How much time?" She smiles bitterly.

He gives her a hug, makes her an appointment with a radiation oncologist and a follow-up visit here in two weeks. I'll be gone by then.

I reach out to touch her shoulder and she hugs me for a minute, awkwardly, my stethocope getting in the way.

"How were the blackberries?" she asks, through tears.

"They—they were great." I'm not sure what to add. "I made a pie," I say, a little shyly.

She nods.

"Thank you," she says.

For what? I wonder. I haven't done anything.

IT'S LUNCHTIME. I want to eat. Suddenly I want to be fat, to shield myself with layers of flesh against wasting, death, destruction.

"You've got a good appetite," my attending comments, watching me gulp down a slice of leftover blackberry pie.

"I think it's my fear of death," I say.

He looks at me strangely.

"Just a joke," I say feebly, although it wasn't.

IN BED THAT night I feel my lymph nodes, moving slowly from my neck to my armpits to my groin. They are all small and normal in consistency. I check over and over, searching for the harbinger of doom. Of course I don't find it; and of course, this is no guarantee that someday it won't come. Over days and weeks the fear fades, but her pleading eyes still haunt me.

39. Tattoo

He's a follow-up patient in the Oncology clinic. The attending glances at the chart as we walk in. "He's doing great," he says. "Prostate cancer ten years ago, we caught it early, no recurrence. He just drops in every year or so for a check."

I talk with him. He's doing fine. I examine his head and neck. "Let me just have a listen here—" I reach to lift his shirt.

He blocks my hand. "Did he warn you?"

"Warn me about what?"

"My tattoo."

"No," I say.

He sighs. "He really should've warned you. Well.... It's okay, I guess. Go ahead."

I study his face but can't read his expression.

I've seen a lot of tattoos in my medical career. Dragons, eagles, hearts, snakes, knives. Vets covered in coarse greenish markings no longer recognizable. More naked women than I could begin to count. I've seen love notes and hate messages, the occasional swastika. I've come to accept men's sheepish faces over the most egregious as a mute apology.

But I've never had anyone warn me about a tattoo.

Trying to imagine how anything could be worse than what I've already seen, I rather gingerly lift his shirt. "Oh, dear . . ." he murmurs. I school my expression to attentive neutrality.

I cannot describe what I see on his chest. I am momentarily stunned, then gulp back—a laugh.

It's—well, it's a bull. But not just any bull. It's sort of a Far Side bull. A sparse, boxy outline of a face, two dots for eyes, a flat, uneven line of a mouth that neither smiles nor frowns. The barest curve of a neck and scrawny shoulders. The bull is huge, its horns stretching across the full span of his chest—yes, horns, also sketched in irregular straight lines, not quite even over his chest, tilting just enough to look off-kilter but not enough to look deliberately so. The ends of each horn are filled in, otherwise the whole sketch is in outline.

The overall effect is of a very large, fairly crooked bull head, its expression somewhere between stunned, confused, and merely very stupid. For reasons that I can't explain but that any follower of Gary Larson understands, it is absolutely hysterical.

"Where'd you get that?" I inquire, as soon as I regain my voice.

"Did it myself," he says, a grin finally bursting out from behind his impenetrable gaze. "I was fourteen. Did it with a needle and some dye and—man, did it hurt. But not half so much as what my mother did to me when she caught me doing it. . . . I was right there." He points to one of the bull's irregular shoulders. "I wasn't quite done. You see, it's higher than the other—"

I nod, as seriously as I can manage.

"That—that is certainly something," I say.

"Isn't it awful?" He twinkles.

"Actually I think it's the funniest thing I've ever seen," I say.

"No," he protests.

"Yes," I say. "Really."

"Thanks," he says, as he puts his shirt back on and prepares to head down the hallway, marking off another cancer-free year.

"No," I say. "Thank you. You take care of that artwork of yours."

"I will," he promises.

40. Who's Mary?

Halfway through my third year, I was pulled from a Gastroenterology elective to spend a week in the ICU covering for a resident who had just had a baby.

Our first call night was long and busy. We admitted half a dozen people, most of them very sick, a few not. The ICU service shares overdose patients with Neurology and Medicine. We got two that night, both healthy young women with serious social problems—homeless, with young children, no money, no marketable skills. They had both taken overdoses of blood pressure medications, obtained who knows where, and needed to be monitored overnight to make sure their blood pressure and heart rhythms stayed okay. The psychiatrists saw them both and felt they didn't need psych hospitalization. By morning the medicines would be cleared from the bloodstream, and they would be free to go.

In fact, it would be more than that. They would be forced to go. The hospital was full, desperate for beds for people who were sick, and nobody who was well enough to go could stay a moment longer than necessary.

I was facing the bleary eyes of my intern, Eric, who like me had been up all night.

"She doesn't want to go," he said. We had just finished rounding on the sicker people, and were now going to take care of discharging these two.

"She doesn't?" Nobody is ever ambivalent about leaving the hospital. There are the people who never want to be there, and the ones who never want to leave.

"It sucks, throwing people out," he said.

"Yes."

"I mean—leaving cynicism aside for a second—poor woman. Her life sucks. And then she takes a bottle of pills in this grand gesture, probably not wanting to die, but asking for help. And then, what do we do? Put her in a bed overnight and throw her on the street."

"I know it sucks, Eric. It really does. But the system's broken, and you and I can't fix it, not this morning, anyway. We can only do the best we can."

"Which is, out on the street."

I sighed. "Well, not exactly. She's homeless with kids, so we can get her a bed at one of the respite houses. She can stay there at least a few days, and they've got social workers to get her started on the next steps. And we can get her an appointment next week with Psychiatry, to work on her depression. It's not much, but it's not quite putting her on the street."

"It'll sound like it to her."

"Maybe. We'll do the best we can. Call Social Work, and get them working on the respite bed. Then we'll go talk to her."

WE WALKED IN together and Eric pulled up a chair while I sat on the bed.

"How are you doing?" I asked.

"Okay, I guess."

"I know you still feel pretty crummy."

She nodded.

"He said I was going to have to leave." She gestured to Eric.

I sighed. "That's something we wanted to talk to you about. What happens next."

"I'm not ready to leave," she said. "I need some time. I need to think things through, get my life in order."

I nodded. "I understand. And those are such important things." Now it's about to get hard, because I'm going to have to reconcile what I think she needs with the reality of what I can offer.

"The problem is, the hospital's not a place where you can do that. I know—" She's taking a breath, and I know what she's about to say. "You think it should be, and actually I think so, too. I wish this were a place where you could come and we could get you back on your feet. But it isn't. We're only set up to deal with a certain kind of problem, acute medical problems that need to be diagnosed and treated. You have a different kind of problem, and we can't fix that here. Partly because we don't have the resources to do it, and partly because we don't have enough room for the people we *can* treat, so nobody who could possibly leave can stay. In a way that's good for you; the hospital's a bad place to be if you don't need it. You get exposed to all kinds of nasty stuff here, and it's best to be somewhere else if you can."

By now she's looking completely dejected.

"But there are some things we can do. We've found a place for you in a respite house, where they look after people who don't need the hospital but need somewhere to go. You can stay there for a little while, while you're sorting things out. They have social workers who are experts in just your kind of situation, and they will help you sort out the steps you can take next. All those questions you asked us earlier—how you're going to get a job and how you'll take care of the kids—those are things they can help you with."

She looks a little brighter, but still uncertain. "You can do it," I say. "You're strong. Look at everything you've done." I'm reaching for details of our conversation in the middle of the night, when we admitted her. I have her slightly mixed up with the other one, the other overdose patient—they were so much alike! Yet I'm remembering more about her story as we talk. There was an abusive boyfriend she'd recently left, an alcohol habit she kicked a few years ago. I have almost all of the details now, although, irritatingly, the one thing I can't come up with is her name.

"You got yourself and your kids out of that bad relationship. You got off the alcohol, and stayed off, in spite of everything that was going on. Those are huge accomplishments." I mean this; I wish that she could see how true it is.

She nods with a little more confidence.

"If you could do that, you can do this next piece. It's going to be hard, but there will be people to help you, and you can do it. We'll get you set up with people who can help, social workers and a psychiatrist for the depression and a medical doctor, too, although luckily your body got through last night without any damage. You're going to be okay. You can do it. I have faith in you—"

Why can't I think of her name? Mary! That was it, Mary. But I mumble it a little.

"I have faith in you, Mary; you can do this."

She nods.

"You're going to be okay."

She nods again.

"Okay?"

"Okay," she says.

We walk out of the room. We're halfway down the hall when Eric can no longer contain his laughter.

"That was really great, but—who's Mary?" he asks.

"What?"

"Mary. You said Mary. I swear you did."

With sinking heart, I wait for the words I know are coming.

"That wasn't Mary. Mary is the other one."

I FOUND AN excuse to go back before she left, and called her by her proper name. I'll always hope she didn't notice, or thought that she misheard me. The strange thing is that, even though I was trying to get her to leave the hospital, and even though I got her name wrong, I really meant my speech.

To this day, whenever I see Eric, now long graduated from the program, he calls me Mary.

41. Rite of Passage

She's seventeen.

Seventeen years old, and coming in for her first Pap smear. I try to remember how old I was, when I had mine. About the same age, I think. Can that be only ten years ago? It seems like forever.

She has shoulder-length brown hair in a ponytail, and bright, round dark brown eyes. She glances around the exam room nervously, as if examining a torture chamber, but her manner is calm.

I review the intake form she's filled out. She's had one sexual partner, she has no symptoms she's concerned about, she's mostly here because she wants to start on the pill.

She clears her throat after we've discussed the intake form. "One other thing—"

"Yes?" I wait while she pauses. A number of expressions flit across her face, some childish, some adult. I can almost see her shifting from moment to moment between the girl she has been and the young woman she is becoming. Adolescents are wonderful this way, fascinating in their contradictions.

"I'm here—without my parents' knowledge," she says rather grandly, drawing herself up straight.

I nod. "Okay. We're used to that. We'll make sure not to send any mail, or call."

"It's okay," she says. "I mean—I think they'd be okay with it. I mean, they know I'm having sex. Well"—now her voice gets a little higher and less measured, more of a little-girl voice—"they thought I was having sex like a year ago! I mean, really! It's only been three months. . . ."

Ah, the outrage! I suppress my smile.

"We'll be careful not to send anything," I say. "You can decide if you're comfortable talking about it with them, and when, and how."

She nods.

I look again at her form. "You're not using anything for protection now?"

"Well—" She pauses. "We were using condoms. We're not—we haven't done anything for a while."

"Okay," I say.

"My boyfriend—" She pauses. "My . . . partner?"

"Partner" is the word used on the intake form, which some people find comfortable and others don't. I flash back suddenly to being in college and having my boyfriend ask about my visit to the doctor. "Did they ask about me?" he wanted to know. "A little," I said. "What did they call me?" We were very concerned with how to name each other in those days. "Boyfriend" seemed too childish, "lover" too explicit, "significant other" too cumbersome. "My 'partner,'" I told him. "Partner?" he protested, scrunching up his nose. "It sounds like we're playing tennis!"

"'Boyfriend' is fine," I tell her. "Whatever word you want to use."

"He's—he's at college. He's coming home for the holidays. That's why I'm here."

"Okay," I say. "That's fine.

I explain the pelvic exam to her, using the little plastic models we keep in the exam room. She listens seriously, wide-eyed, asks several questions. She is a model of deliberate composure; I can sense the fear coursing through her, and her absolute determination not to give in to it.

I feel a strong rush of protectiveness and admiration. I almost wish she'd let go a little, so I could comfort her. Her stoicism holds her somewhat outside the range of consolation. At the same time, I have immense respect for her solitary courage.

The exam goes fine. I've worked hard at learning to do a painless speculum exam, motivated by my own bad experiences. She's terrific.

She doesn't flinch. She's even able to relax the muscles I tell her to relax, a difficult feat that makes the whole process much easier. I explain each thing I'm doing as I do it, and ask frequently how she's doing. She says "Okay" in a clear voice untinged by panic.

After the Pap, I hesitate over cultures. "We check routinely for STDs, unless you specifically want us not to."

She shrugs. "You can if you want, if it makes you feel better." I smile at this phrasing, her rather airy acknowledgment of my agenda. "But, it won't. . . . It was. . . ." She drops her voice a little, shyly. "It was the first time for both of us."

"Okay." I send the cultures anyway. I trust her word, but I'm not taking chances on his. She's right. It does make me feel better.

The whole thing is over in a few minutes. "You can get dressed now," I say.

"That wasn't bad at all!" she announces, hopping off the exam table, her whole body exuding relief.

"I told you it wouldn't hurt," I say, feeling more than a little relieved myself.

AFTER SHE'S DRESSED, I come back in and we go over information about birth control pills. With the exam over she is noticeably more relaxed, chatty, cheerful. I can measure her anxiety about the exam more clearly by the dramatic change in its absence than by anything she displayed at the time.

"What are your plans for next year?" I ask. She's a senior.

"I'm waiting to hear from colleges," she says. "I mean—I'll go, I just don't know where yet. I'm at one of those high schools where everybody goes to college, but everyone's all competitive about where. God forbid you should go to a *state* school or something. It's ridiculous."

She shudders half jokingly, and again I feel her hovering on that line between youth and maturity. Part of her is able to see all the competition as silly, but not enough that she wouldn't be crushed if she didn't get into the college of her choice.

"Where do you want to go?" I ask.

"Well, it's all complicated," she says, sighing. "See, my boyfriend—he's at Penn. So he's like Mr. Smart Guy." She rolls her eyes, and I grin. "So now there's all this pressure on me, you see?" She looks up in appeal. "I applied early to Williams, I'm really hoping I get in, but I don't know. . . ."

We talk about Penn, and Williams, for a few minutes. She's animated, cheerful, opinionated. Then she suddenly spins on me, her face dawning with a new suspicion. "Wait—where did *you* go?"

"Me? I went to Yale," I admit.

"Oh, my God!" she shrieks, burying her head in her hands.

"What?" I ask, startled.

"Now you're intimidating." She pouts at me.

"I'm sorry," I say.

"Well, before, you weren't intimidating, when I thought you could have gone to—" She breaks off.

"Podunk U?" I suggest. She hangs her head.

"Where did you go to med school?" she demands. Then adds quickly, "I'm sorry—is that too personal?"

I'm amused by her thinking a piece of information I put on my office wall is personal, when many of my patients seem to feel quite comfortable asking if I'm married, dating, planning to have kids, and all manner of prying.

"Dartmouth," I say.

"Dartmouth!" Her eyes light up. "I applied to Dartmouth. Did you like it?"

"I loved it," I say. "It's so beautiful up there. . . ."

"I've heard—I don't know. Both some great things, and some not so great ones. . . ."

"We didn't interact with the undergraduate school much," I say. "I've heard it's kind of an old-boys' network, but I don't really know."

She raises her eyebrows. "An old-boys' network—as opposed to Yale?"

She draws the word out, teasingly, to two syllables: Yay-uhl.

I shrug and smile.

Finally I send her off, with a pack of pills, a return appointment in a few months, a number to call if she has any questions or problems.

"Thank you," she says, offering me her hand, a little stiffly. Her manner is again very adult. "I—I thought this would be hard, and it really wasn't."

"I'm glad," I say, really meaning it. "Good luck."

"Thank you," she says, and walks away, her stride confident and resolute.

42. Crixivan

It's a routine follow-up visit for a man with HIV. He's come in for the usual blood tests, medication refills, and a quick hello. He's doing well, tolerating his triple therapy regimen with no serious side effects, managing to juggle all the pills. He mentions he's going to be traveling, and asks about his crixivan, a drug that needs to be kept refrigerated. He'd like a prescription for the liquid form, which is more stable at warm temperatures and therefore simpler for travelers.

I reach for the prescription pad. As I tear off his script, I add: "Actually, you probably don't need one. Usually if it's the same drug they'll substitute any formulation. Most pharmacists are pretty good about that."

"Oh, I have a great pharmacist," he says.

"That's important, especially with a condition like this one—"

"I've known my pharmacist for years," he says. "He's a terrific guy. Smart, friendly, very helpful." He smiles. "Actually—this is kind of a funny story. When I first starting taking the antiretrovirals . . ." He pauses, as if not quite sure how much to tell. "Well, I'd known him all this time, but he had no idea that I was gay, much less HIV positive."

"Wow." It suddenly occurs to me how much pharmacists must know about their patients' lives. I've always known how much information you can get from a med list. Our computer system gives a full record, with dates, and you can read in it the story line of a patient's history—another antibiotic and decongestant, likely a round of sinusitis; a steroid taper suggests a flare of asthma if they're on inhalers, arthritis if they're on nonsteroidals, maybe inflammatory bowel disease if they're on salsalate—and so on. Everything from cancer to mental illness to impotence, not to mention HIV, has telltale signs on a med list.

And of course the pharmacists can read that better than I can. As a doctor I'm supposed to know, and I get to discuss it all with the patient, whereas the pharmacist doesn't necessarily have such an easy forum. That must be a difficult position for them.

"So," my patient is continuing, "when I first started on the HIV meds, I went in to pick them up; and he was standing there, all, well, long-faced and sad-looking. Even a little teary . . ."

He smiles wistfully, remembering the poignant moment.

"So, we went in the back and had a long talk." He shakes his head a few times, smiles. "I think he's dealing with it okay now."

He stands up, waves his script. "Thanks a lot, Doc; I'll see you in a couple months."

"Sure," I say.

43. God Rest His Soul

I walk in to see my first patient on Friday morning in the Women's Clinic. The schedule says she's here for an annual exam and Pap smear, referred by her regular physician, a rheumatologist.

She's older than most of the patients we see here—seventy, I calculate, glancing down at her chart. Her white hair is teased. She's just a little plump, sitting rather primly on her chair with her legs crossed. The clinic's new-patient form is in her lap, and she is intently studying the questions.

With the help of the form, I run through her past medical history, her current problems. She's been mostly healthy, and it sounds like the rheumatologist has her primary care issues well under control.

"I've been going to him for fifteen years," she says. "He's a wonderful man."

"He certainly is," I say. "I've worked with him."

"I know he's supposed to just be a joint doctor," she says. "But he takes care of everything I need done—except this, of course."

I have her change into a gown, then I come back to do the breast exam and Pap smear.

"You've been through this before," I say. "So you know what it's like. But I'll explain everything as I do it. I want you to let me know if anything I do hurts or makes you uncomfortable."

She sighs as she clambers onto the examining table. "I hate it," she says.

"We all hate it," I say, sighing. "But I'll try to make it as comfortable as possible."

"The last time—" she says. "It was a couple years ago. I came into the clinic, and the doctor was a young man, with wild, long curly hair. I look down between my legs, and all I can see is this man's head. . . ."

She shivers.

"It's all fine for you young women, I suppose," she says. "I'm sure you don't care about things like that. But when you get to be my age—it just doesn't sit right. So I asked them if they could schedule me with a woman this time."

"Actually," I say, "I don't know how much it has to do with age. I'd just as soon have a woman doctor, too. For some things, anyway."

She nods.

After the exam, I step out to let her put her clothes on. When I come back in, she's bent over the intake form again.

"This is mostly intended for . . . younger women, isn't it?"

"I suppose," I say. I'd never really thought about it. "Most of the patients who come through this clinic are younger."

"There are lots of, questions about sex, and things," she says.

I nod. She'd told me earlier that she hadn't been sexually active since her husband died, some years before. I feel like she's going somewhere with this line of questioning, but I can't figure out where.

With an air of sudden resolve, she points to a word on the form. "What is this, 'trichomonas'?"

I blink, caught off guard by the unexpected question and the strange intensity in her tone. "Trichomonas? It's a sexually transmitted disease. It's fairly common, causes a variety of symptoms—"

She stops me. "When you say, sexually transmitted—" She pauses. "That means, if you get it, you must have gotten it from someone."

"Yes," I say, slowly beginning to understand.

"And he must have gotten it from someone else."

"Yes," I admit, very quietly.

I watch her face carefully, not sure of what I've just done, not knowing what is going to happen next. Her brows are deeply furrowed, her lips move a little, as if framing words she can't quite get out. But then she just nods, slowly and thoughtfully.

"God rest his soul," she murmurs at last.

"Are you okay?" I ask after a moment.

There's a pause.

"Yes," she says. She looks up, gives her hands a quick shake as if pulling herself together. "Well. I—I thought that's what it meant. But I was never sure." Suddenly she smiles wryly. "I'm glad I asked you. I've waited since 1949 to ask a doctor that question."

"Oh," I say.

"That's when they told me I had that, trichomonas."

"I'm sorry," I say.

She shrugs. "Well—it's all so long ago. He's dead now."

I nod.

"But I did wonder. There was no one—he was the only one I ever . . ."

"I understand," I say.

But of course I don't, not really. What would it be like to be seventy years old and learn that the only man you'd ever made love to had cheated on you?

She stands up from the chair, shakes my hand, and says, "Thank you." I watch as she walks down the hallway, her teased white hair bouncing a little with the movement of her plump body, a picture of prim efficiency, of determined calm.

44. We Loved You

The Neurology resident looks stressed, flipping irritably through her patient cards. "Okay, who do we have. . . . There's a bunch of people who have been here for a while—all pretty stable. A couple of overdoses who came in last night. And then there's this one guy upstairs who's sick as shit."

The attending raises his eyebrows, and the resident flushes. "Well, he is," she says. "Found unconscious, head trauma. No one knows how long he was out before someone found him, outside in a garbage dumpster. He's up in the ICU on a vent, barely holding on."

The three of us are standing in the Neurology team room, getting ready to make morning rounds. I don't say anything, just sip my coffee and try to suppress my irritation at being here. I'm in the middle of a third-year clinic month, a nice interlude of no call and free weekends. I had planned to spend this lovely May Saturday sailing on Lake Washington in a friend's boat. Then I got the call. I was being pulled in to cover for a Neurology intern who was going to the yearly interns' retreat.

This sort of thing would be less painful if there were some kind of compensation for it, i.e., extra pay, an extra weekday off, whatever. Instead it's just thirty-six extra hours at the hospital playing an intern for the Neurology service, a role I hated when I actually was an intern, and which hasn't grown on me in the intervening two years. The fact that both of my best friends are spending the weekend in San Francisco, having begged out of similar duty by saying they had airline tickets, does not make me more cheerful. "Airline tickets," I think to myself bitterly. "I'll have to remember that for next time."

I try not to dwell on this, without much success, as I stand blearily drinking coffee and listening to the Neuro resident talk about the patients on the service. I console myself by thinking that it should be pretty easy for me at this stage to do an intern's job. I'll just do scut work and leave anything serious to the resident, try to get through the day without really having to wake up.

"We'd better see the guy in the ICU first," the Neuro resident says, looking haggard. She fills in the details as we walk up the stairs. He's about thirty, he was found downtown in a dumpster very early this morning. He barely had a pulse initially, coded briefly in the ER, is still pretty unstable in terms of blood pressure and oxygen. The bigger problem is his head. His skull was smashed with a blunt object, presumably by whoever threw him in the dumpster. A large part of his brain was destroyed in the initial injury, and what's left is rapidly giving in to swelling and inflammation and lack of blood supply. The only indication that he isn't brain dead is that his body occasionally takes a breath on its own without the ventilator. This means that his brain stem, the old, deep part of the brain that controls basic reflexes like breathing, isn't completely gone.

That's all the good news there is, and it isn't much.

As we walk into his room, the nurse looks up. "The family just arrived," she says. "They're waiting for you in the conference room."

"I heard there wasn't a family," the resident says.

"It's complicated," the nurse answers.

The attending glances at his watch. "We really need to round. We'll just say hi to them quickly and come back later."

"He's estranged from the family," the nurse says. "They haven't had any contact in three years."

THE THREE OF US—the attending, the Neuro resident, and I—walk into the ICU conference room. There's a long, broad table in the middle of the room. I notice immediately the arrangement of the people around it. On the right side, centered on the long axis of the table, is a trio of figures. Sitting in the middle is an African-American woman, in her sixties, heavyset, in a silk dress and heels. She chose formal clothes for the hospital, at this early hour on a Saturday morning. The mother. Her eyes are dry but red, and her mascara is smeared. She has been crying, but has chosen not to cry in front of us.

She is flanked by two men. On the near side is a young man in his thirties, tall with a muscular build. He too has been crying, and he keeps one arm curled protectively around his mother. Her other son. On the woman's far side is a man of intermediate age, perhaps midforties. He sits stiffly and looks uncomfortable, his eyes wandering around the room. A cousin, perhaps.

On the left side of the table, another man sits alone. He is white, with bleached spiked hair, rail thin. His arms are tattooed, and his jean jacket is scruffy but clean. He keeps his eyes fixed on the table, except when someone is talking. Then he watches them intently.

We sit down—the attending at the head of the long table, the resident and I on either side of him. He clears his throat and begins to talk.

"I understand you know more or less what's been going on."

They nod uncertainly.

"He's very sick. Right now his heart is very unstable. There's also been brain damage."

The mother chokes, a stifled sob, and there's a pause as the son quiets her.

What, I wonder, estranges a man from his family for three years? Sexuality? Drugs? Religion? Was it the son or the family that made the choice, or both—or was it one of those terrible situations in which everyone feels backed into an unintended path? I look at the lone man on the far side—clearly apart from the family, clearly a friend from more recent years. Was he a lover, a comrade in addiction or in recovery, an ally in some lifestyle or belief? I find no answers in the downcast eyes, the thin but friendly face.

How did the man in the next room end up with his head crushed in, in a dumpster? I'll never know. Strangely, I'm less curious about that than the dynamics in this room. I'll fight the losing battle for him, but he's going to die. The aftermath will be for the living.

The attending is finishing his short, dry speech. "We don't know. We'll do everything we can."

We file out, leaving the four of them in their seats. I wonder if words between them will follow, but I doubt it. The wall across the middle of the room was invisible but strong.

"Well," the attending says, "let's get back to rounds."

We round for a painful hour and a half. I wonder, why should I get to know these people? I'm here for twenty-four hours. I don't need to hear about three young patients in persistent vegetative states to remind me how depressing this service is. We end up back in the ICU.

His blood pressure is dropping even lower now.

"Looks crummy," the attending comments.

"Yeah."

"Well, do your thing. Good luck." He glances back from the doorway. "Looks like he could use a Swan."

THE SWAN-GANZ catheter is a mainstay of critical care monitoring. It's a balloon attached to a long wire, which is inserted through a thick catheter into the jugular vein. You ease it forward by feeding the wire into the vein, monitoring the balloon's location in the bloodstream through a pressure gauge on its tip. There's a certain pressure pattern in the vein, which changes as the balloon moves into the atrium of the heart, then again as it floats into the ventricle. Carrying the wire along, it finally passes out of the heart, into the pulmonary artery, yet another pattern. You continue feeding the wire, letting it ease forward until the pressure pattern changes one more time, as the balloon wedges into a small vein in the lung.

Once the catheter is in place, a huge amount of information can be gained from it. You can make precise measurements of the pressures and flow in the heart and the lungs, gleaning information about the workings of both the right and left side of the heart, and about the flow of blood and movement of oxygen and carbon dioxide across the lung. Otherwise, these things can't be precisely measured. A Swan is a tremendous resource in the care of someone very ill.

A Swan is tricky to place. First, there's getting the thick catheter into the jugular vein, a complex task in its own right. Then, as you insert the balloon, you have to identify each pattern quickly and correctly—if you get to the wrong place or go too far, the consequences can be terrible. Theoretically, moving the balloon through the heart is easy. The balloon is carried by the blood and follows the blood flow to the place where you want it to be. In practice, it's not so simple. There's a tendency for the wire to get caught or tangled in the heart's ventricle, and it takes some finesse to get it through. Finally—just to make things interesting—the tip of the wire can tickle the heart as it moves through, making it fire off extra beats and go into abnormal rhythms. Occasionally, the heart can stop completely—this has happened to me twice.

This process is poetically called "floating a Swan." Drs. Swan and Ganz were the two men who invented it; there's no relation to the bird. It's a flowery term for a medical procedure performed almost always under desperate circumstances. On the other hand, there is something magical about floating a balloon through someone's heart. Once I did one under fluoroscopy, a special kind of real-time X-ray that lets you actually watch the wire and balloon move. It was terrifying. It was technically easier but psychologically much harder than floating one the usual way, by rhythm. I had to face what I was really doing. It wasn't just a concept or a metaphor. I was actually wriggling an object through a beating heart.

THE NEURO RESIDENT looks green as the attending disappears. She glances sidelong toward me. It occurs to me that she's not comfortable dealing with this, that she wants me to take over. Oh, come on, I want to say. I'm playing the intern. You're playing the senior. I don't want to switch roles.

I'm being unfair to her, of course. She's in her second year of training, and I'm in my third. I remember her vaguely from last year, a wide-eyed intern. That wasn't so very long ago. Besides, as a Medicine trainee, I'm much more experienced in critical care than they are in Neuro.

I feel the mindless day of simple scut work slipping from my hands. Looks like I'll have to wake up after all. I swallow the dregs of my coffee.

"I have two consults to do," she says, a little desperately. "Do you think you could just? . . ."

Don't "just" me, I want to say. Yes, I can handle this guy and his Swan and everything else for you, and yes, I'm going to, particularly since I'm better trained for it than you are. And no, it's not your fault that I'm not basking on the deck of a sailboat in the middle of Lake Washington. But don't "just" me when you know this fiasco is a lot more difficult than your two consults.

"Sure," I say.

Two hours later, I leave his bedside for the first time. The Swan is in, a tiny balloon on a wire wrapped through his heart—I don't pause to wonder at this, there's too much else to do. I've been tweaking his three drips of vasopressors and adjusting his fluids and his ventilator settings and every other minute detail. I run to Radiology to look at the latest chest film, and the radiologist says, "Do you understand how shitty this looks?"

"Yeah," I say. "Actually, I'm amazed we haven't coded him yet."

At that moment my pager goes off, and I say, "I suspect this means we'll be doing it soon." Before I have time to dial, the overhead announces the code: 9 East, his floor, and then his room number.

I run the nine flights and burst into his room, breathless. I find a strange sight. The code is under way, and the room is full of senior residents in Medicine. Of course. All of them, like me, have been called in to cover interns at the retreat.

Codes are always stressful, perhaps the ultimate stressful moment. Each of us, in our final year of hospital-based training, is as comfortable with them as we'll ever be. Today, instead of one of us directing our interns and carrying most of the weight of the responsibility, we're all here together, we can share.

I take charge—he's my patient, after all. Someone is doing compressions, and someone is calling out the rhythm from the heart monitor. Each time I call for a drug, someone has anticipated my needs and has it waiting. The code takes on a certain social tone. I call out, "Clear for shock," and everyone says, "Clear." The moment after the shock, someone says, reading the monitor, "V-tach," and someone else says, "I really like your new haircut."

We have just got him back into a decent though wavery rhythm when the code pagers go off again—someone else's patient, this time.

"Go ahead," I say. "I've got this." And everyone disperses.

Within a few minutes, we're back to where we started. He's stabilized for the moment, but still hanging on by only a thread. Worse, the nurses tell me that since I went down to Radiology he hasn't taken a breath on his own.

"Someone needs to talk to the family."

I nod, glance instinctively around the room. The attending isn't here. The Neuro resident didn't even come up for the code. There's no one who could go but me.

"I'll be out there in a second."

THE SOCIAL WORKER and one of the nurses are in the room, talking with the mother, brother, and cousin. The friend is gone. They fall silent as I walk in, something which still feels strange to me: that I should be the one that they were waiting for, the bearer of the awaited news, the one whose role is so important that they go quiet to hear me say my piece, then let me go quickly back to caring for their son, brother, cousin.

I sit down, acutely aware of my movements, gestures, words.

"As the nurses have told you, his heart stopped a few minutes ago. With the help of medications and electric shock, we were able to get it started again. However, his blood pressure is still extremely low, and he is having difficulty keeping enough oxygen in his blood." I look at them, judging whether this is sinking in, and they each nod, slowly.

"Also, you remember that we told you earlier that he was taking breaths in addition to the ventilator, and that this was a sign that some part of his brain was still functioning. Unfortunately, he stopped taking those extra breaths a little while ago, which leaves us without any sign that his brain is working."

I take a deep breath. "These are not good signs," I say. "I don't want to frighten you, but I want you to understand that this is very, very serious.

I can't offer you much hope. But we are continuing to do everything that we possibly can for him."

They nod.

"Do you have any questions?" I wait a long moment, knowing questions can take a long time to formulate into words. But they all shake their heads. I nod, stand, and go back to the patient's room.

STEPPING FROM A family meeting into the room of a sick ICU patient is like diving from air into water: the physical distance is so small, yet everything about the two worlds is intensely different. The thick emotional soup of the family meeting—the importance of each word and tone and gesture, the paramount need to correctly read and transmit subtle signals—gives way to the icy depersonalization of the patient's room, a complete ban enforced on all questions of content and meaning, context and emotion. There isn't room for those here.

Standing in the room I do not see his mangled face, his swollen, bloody lips. I don't see the tattoo on his chest or even its muscles as I assess the rise and fall of his ribs with the breaths of the ventilator. I stare at him and see the X-ray on the board downstairs, the numbers and graphs on the vent and the computer and the wall monitor. He is not the estranged son of the family in the next room. He is a puzzle to be solved. He is physics and physiology.

Both of these worlds are familiar to me, comfortable in their way. I can hold a family member's hands and listen for the breathing change that shows they are about to cry. I can touch a shoulder and feel a grieving body shift its weight out toward my hand. And I can manage vents and float Swan-Ganz catheters and interpret arterial blood gasses. In some perhaps twisted way, I enjoy both these things, but the magnitude of the transition will never cease to surprise and shock me.

AN HOUR LATER he codes again, and fifteen minutes later, a third time. We get him back each time, but he's slipping. We call this neurogenic shock, meaning that if the brain is injured badly enough, the body just shuts down. We're doing everything we can, and it isn't enough.

I gather the family again, in a lounge this time, a smaller, more comfortable room.

"I'm sorry," I say. "I wish that there were something else I could say. But he's dying."

There's a silent pause as the mother slumps into her older son.

"His heart has stopped twice in the last half hour. We're using all the machines and medicines we have, and his blood pressure and his oxygen aren't high enough to keep his body alive. He's going, fast, and we can't stop it."

After a long time, the mother nods. "I want to see him," she says.

I nod.

The brother draws a breath to speak. He, unlike his mother, had gone in to the bedside earlier. He didn't stay long. I can't blame him. His brother's face is a pulverized mess, a giant purple bruise; his eyes aren't visible through all the swelling. There are tubes coming out of him everywhere. His only movement is the mechanical rise and fall of the ventilator.

"Mom," he begins.

At that moment the nurse raps sharply on the door. "Now," she says. and I turn to follow her.

The code pagers ring out again. This time there is no chatter about haircuts, and the combined strength of all of us isn't enough to get him back.

SHE KNOWS; I can see it in her eyes as I walk back in—or perhaps she can see it in mine.

"It's over," she says, and I nod.

"I'm sorry."

She doesn't speak, holds the tears inside. "I want to see him."

I nod again.

The nurses have been busy, pulling out the tubes, putting away the machines. They've wiped the blood from his face and lifted a clean blanket to his chin.

She stays quiet as she walks to the bedside, though her face is streaming now with tears. She touches his bruised, not yet cold forehead, traces his eyebrow and his swollen cheekbone.

She begins to whisper, and then to scream.

"James. We still loved you, James. We did. We *did*. My baby, my baby . . . We loved you. *We still loved you. . . .*"

Her oldest finally reaches out and draws her into his arms.

"He knows, Mama. He *knows.*"

I have been hovering in the back of the room, wondering if I could soothe or help, but I feel I have intruded, violated, simply by witnessing this much.

I slip away, leaving them alone. Her voice does not fade from my ears.

OVERNIGHT THE NEURO resident and I admit a handful of folks, the usual Neuro stuff. An older woman with a stroke, weak on the left side but stable—she'll recover almost fully. A young man with his first seizure—the usual drill, a head CT, labs, seizure medications. And a handful of intentional and accidental drug overdoses, intubated in the field for respiratory arrest. They'll be physically fine by morning, ready to be reviewed by the psychiatrists.

I sleep for an hour or two, wake up at five, and start my own little rounds. I walk through the ICU with a respiratory tech extubating all the overdoses. They cough and sputter and breathe and I write their progress notes. By seven my work is done. As the attending and the resident walk into the team room to round, I hand them a fistful of notes. It isn't clear from the coverage arrangement whether I'm supposed to stay for rounds, but I've decided not to.

"Everybody's doing fine," I say. They already know about the dead one.

"It's nice having a senior Medicine resident around," the attending says. "You're welcome anytime."

"I'll remember that," I say, and force myself not to run until the door closes behind me.

*   *   *

AN HOUR LATER I meet my friend at his boat dock. We hoist the boat's sails and coast in silence into the water. I squint into the dazzling light, the clear blue sky, the sun glittering on the water.

"How was your day?" he asks.

"Long," I say. He knows better than to ask more.

I close my eyes and feel the sun against my skin, listen to the light slap and whirl of the water against the hull. The mother's voice still echoes in my ears: *We loved you. . . .* The hospital, faintly visible above the hill, seems light-years away. I can't figure out whether that world is a dream, or this one.

45. Commencement

There is no ceremony to mark the end of residency.

There's a little brunch for the third-years in the last month, and you get a certificate saying you completed the program. I went to the brunch—they had arranged for coverage—then back to the hospital. It was pleasant enough, but lacked the feel of a commencement. It certainly wasn't something you would invite your family to.

It's ironic, because of all the steps along the way—finishing college, finishing medical school—this feels like the biggest accomplishment. Just getting through these years has been the hardest thing I've ever done. Though I came out of medical school with the glorious title "Doctor" and out of residency only with the unwieldy adjunct "Board Eligible in Internal Medicine," the truth is that it was residency, not medical school, that transformed me from a student into a physician.

This is when I want the calls, the kisses on the cheek, the overblown congratulations that rang so strangely false at those previous commencements. "Now," I want to say, "now I have really accomplished something."

But the calls don't come. Next year, I will be staying on at the hospital as a chief resident, a teaching and administrative job, helping to run the program I just finished. Adding a single word to my title, though it changes my life completely, does not attract much attention.

One of the many lessons of residency is that great events can pass with little ceremony, and this one is trivial by comparison to many. So my gym friend Chris and I will rent a canoe and share a tiny bottle of flat Champagne in the middle of the lake, and call it good.

But first I have to finish.

ON MY FINAL call night of residency, I have a brand-new intern, just starting his first week. He is bright-eyed and bushy-tailed and a little bit stunned. I watch him with a strange sense of wonder, remembering myself three years ago. We stick close together, as I try to show him everything from how to handle cross-cover calls to where the bathrooms are. I hear him answering pages: "This is Dr. Tannis. . . ." I note the awe in his voice, the twinkle in his eyes. After he hangs up, I catch him whispering the words again: "Dr. Tannis," softly to himself. He catches my smile and frowns theatrically.

"You're laughing at me."

"No," I say, although he's partly right, I am laughing. I can't explain to him all the thoughts that are going through my mind. I am remembering myself driving across the country on the way from medical school to residency, using "Doc" as my handle on the CB. I remember trying to get used to the idea of that word applied to myself, feeling over and over again the soft thrill of it. I try to recapture that excitement, and also to understand the new feeling that has grown from and beyond it, the confidence that has blossomed as that first wonder faded. What a journey this has been.

I SIT WITH him as he writes orders, glancing over each line as he writes them. I teach him the little details—how much potassium to give for replacement, what dose of antibiotic to choose, how often to check a hematocrit on a GI bleeder—that have become so familiar that I have come to believe people are born knowing them. He makes the same mistakes I made as a new intern: trying to do too much or too little at once, not having the right sense of balance, misprioritizing which problems need to be handled first. He's smart, though, and enthusiastic. He'll turn out fine.

He feels slow and gets frustrated, and I tease him: "Really, you're being too hard on yourself. It takes at least two days to reach your peak efficiency at this job. Give yourself a few more hours."

He looks at me suspiciously, and I stick my tongue out.

"Hey!" he says.

I laugh.

THE EVENING IS busy in a steady, manageable way. After midnight, it gets quiet. I take him down to the call room area. We walk down the long hallway from the hospital into the research building where the call rooms are. His fresh interest makes me acutely aware of the emotions I have built up about this place, the rich and often contradictory layers of feeling. I resent the hospital hierarchy for not finding its residents a place to sleep in the main building, someplace less than a five-minute walk from the patients whose crises we are supposed to manage in the middle of the night. At the same time, I enjoy a secret, shameful pleasure in the same distance, in being far enough away to achieve a psychological distance from the hospital, create a thin mental wall between myself and it.

I show him the little staircase leading to the rooms, make him write down the combination to the door. I show him the lounge, the sofa in front of the television which I used to watch on call nights until I became too frustrated by the constant interruption of my pager. The bathroom where I took fast, edgy showers, always afraid that the code pager would ring and I'd arrive late, dripping, half-dressed. I lead him in to the austere little bedrooms, explain how to adjust the heat and open the windows, all the details I can think of. I show him the refrigerator and the shelf where stale leftover pastries are sometimes put for us. He can't know yet the tortured mixture of gratitude and resentment I feel about those pastries, the pleasure of being fed at all, the anger at its being too little and too late and stale. He'll know these feelings soon enough, too soon.

I save the best for last. When he's seen the rest, I lead him to the door that opens onto a little roof balcony. We walk out gingerly onto the gravelly tarred surface, and I bring him to the edge where you can see the water, the reflections of the houseboat lights sparkling and dancing on the canal.

His attention is elsewhere. "Where does the ladder go?" he asks.

I follow his eyes to a rickety metal ladder running up the wall above the balcony. "I don't know," I say, surprised that I never saw it there before.

He is already gone, disappearing over the top of the next roof up. His head reappears over the top. "Come on."

"Careful of the spider," he cautions as I scramble up the ladder, but I don't see it. I'll discover it on the way down, a huge hairy brown spider with its web laced among the rungs. I've treated brown recluse bites, and I will be frightened, frozen for an instant. On the way up, it is just an unintelligible comment from the intern, another small addition to the countless hazards of residency I have passed safely by without realizing the danger.

The ladder ends on a higher roof, where another leads higher still, and suddenly we are standing on top of the hospital. The city stretches out below us, its familiar hills and valleys, the curves of the lakes and Puget Sound, the downtown skyline. The long dark swath cut by the arboretum, its tall trees lightless in the night.

The most gripping thing is not the view but the birds. There are more seagulls here than I have ever seen away from the ocean, and they are angry. After a few uncertain squawks and swoops on our first appearance, they rise into a concerted frenzy. They fly just barely above us, only a few inches over our heads, in a madly choreographed swirling dance. At first it seems impossible, an unending line of gulls diving at us two by two in rapid succession, breaking apart just over us to fly off into the darkness.

Then I realize they are flying in circles, two loops that intersect above our heads to create the effect of an endless barrage. The pattern is gorgeous and strange and dizzying. The peach-colored lights of the hospital reflect off their white wings and bellies, so they are brightly lit against the black night sky. And they are screaming, individual cries coalescing into a constant steady howl.

I feel as if I were in a movie, a gorgeous scene created to build suspense or mark some critical moment—Hitchcock could have filmed this scene. I cannot quite believe this is happening, or understand why.

"I wonder what's upsetting them?" my intern asks, as if reading my thoughts. His voice sounds small and timid against the screaming of the gulls.

"Not used to having people here, I guess," I say, a little uncertainly.

"Maybe they'd settle if we sat?"

We pick the spot with the best view and sit down, dangling our legs over the edge of the building. Different levels of building and roof stretch below us, the huge chaotic bulk of the hospital complex.

What strange buildings hospitals are. Conceived as grand architectural objects, often; the ultimate public building, this place where we come to give birth and die. But they evolve along more prosaic, utilitarian principles, wings cut and pasted to suit their changing needs. So they end as a hodgepodge of the grand and the practical, a conglomerate of architectural philosophies and styles—a microcosm of the city that they serve.

THE GULLS DO seem happier now that we are sitting. The noise quiets, and the flying spirals stop. After a few minutes, the sky is peaceful again. I look around to a new surprise.

"They're watching us."

The intern follows my gaze, nods slowly. The gulls have settled, a sentry marking each corner of the building, each edge. A number are lined along the walls nearest where we are sitting. They are all quite still, all staring directly at us with dark, round, unintelligible eyes.

Suddenly he points. "What's that?"

"What?"

I peer in the direction he indicates, a dimly lit strip of roof twenty feet below us. At first I see nothing, then my eyes catch a movement.

There is something down there, something small and fuzzy, making anxious stumbling movements. My first thought is that it's a rat, and my toes curl involuntarily. Then I realize, of course, it is a baby seagull.

"No wonder they're so upset. . . ." He breathes softly.

We understand each other, I think, the birds and the doctors. Our roles are not so different. We are both doing our best to protect the weak, the vulnerable of our species. We are quiet now, but vigilant.

I look back down at the city. I wonder where the person is who's waking up now with pain in his chest or his head or his belly. I wonder which set of lights of a car or an ambulance will bring my next admission.

The intern's pager goes off, and with one last, reluctant gaze into the blue-black sky, he turns and climbs back down.

In a minute I will follow him, knowing that I need to be close by in case something happens, in case he needs me. In a minute my own pager will go off, summoning me to the ER, reminding me that the night's not over yet.

Glossary

ABG: arterial blood gas; test run on blood drawn from an artery (typically the radial artery in the wrist) to determine oxygen and carbon dioxide levels

ADENOCARCINOMA: cancer of glandular tissue

A-FIB: atrial fibrillation (*see*)

ALBUTEROL: medication used in aerosolized form to open bronchial airways in asthma or other lung disease

A-LINE: arterial catheter, typically placed in radial artery for continual monitoring of blood pressure and access to arterial blood for oxygen and carbon dioxide monitoring

AMPHO: amphoterocin (*see*)

AMPHOTEROCIN: antifungal medication used for severe fungal infections

AMYLOIDOSIS: poorly understood disorder in which abnormal protein is deposited in multiple organs causing damage to blood vessels and other tissues

ANALGESIC: pain medication

ANGIOGRAM: image of a blood vessel created by shooting radioactive dye into the vessel through a directed catheter, often inserted into an artery in the groin. Commonly done on the blood vessels of the heart (coronary angiogram) or brain (cerebral angiogram)

ANTIBODY: immune molecule that recognizes and attacks a foreign protein (antigen)

ANTIGEN: fragment of a protein recognized by the immune system

ANTIRETROVIRAL: medication used against a class of viruses called retroviruses, including HIV and hepatitis B

ANTIVIRAL: medication used against viruses (HIV, herpes, etc.)

ASCITES: excessive fluid in the abdominal cavity, seen in liver disease and certain cancers and infections

ASCITIC: having to do with ascites (*see*)

ASPERGILLOSIS: infection with the aspergillus fungus

ASPERGILLUS: a type of invasive fungal infection

ASYSTOLE: heart stoppage with absence of electrical activity; "flatline"

ATIVAN: common sedative medication

ATRIAL FIBRILLATION (A-FIB): irregular heartbeat caused by erratic contraction of the atria, the small chambers of the heart; the ventricles (large chambers) contract normally, so, unlike ventricular fibrillation (v-fib), this is not necessarily life threatening

ATTENDING: physician who has completed training in a specialty; used in an academic setting to refer to doctors who are supervising those still in training

BENZODIAZEPENE: common class of sedative medication including Valium, Xanax, and Ativan

BIOPSY: piece of tissue removed from the body for microscopic analysis

BRADY: bradycardia (*see*); also used as a verb, slowing of the heart rate

BRADYCARDIA: abnormally slow heart rate

BRONCHOSCOPY: test in which a small flexible tube is inserted through the nose or mouth into the trachea to allow direct examination and biopsies of the airways

BRONCHOSPASM: closure or tightening of the airways (bronchi), as in asthma or COPD (*see*)

CACHECTIC: excessively thin

CANNULA: stiff catheter (*see*), often used as a guide for placing a longer, softer catheter into a vein

CARCINOID: a rare type of tumor, generally found in the lung or gastrointenstinal tract, that secretes serotonin and related hormones, causing diffuse symptoms including flushing, high blood pressure, and diarrhea

CARCINOMA: cancerous tissue

CATHETER: tube placed into a body space, including the bladder (Foley catheter), vein, spinal column, etc.

CC: milliliter

CCU: Cardiac Intensive Care Unit

CELLULITIS: infection of the deep layers of the skin

CENTRAL LINE: large IV catheter placed into one of the large veins near the heart, commonly the jugular or subclavian vein in the neck or the femoral vein in the groin. Allows rapid infusion of drugs, fluid, or blood, as well as monitoring of pressure in the veins

CEPHALOSPORIN: a class of antibiotic

CNA: certified nursing assistant

COAGULATION: clotting of the blood

CODE: the process of attempting to revive a patient after sudden death (cardiopulmonary arrest) occurs, following the protocols of advanced cardiac life support (ACLS). As a verb, "to code," either (for a patient) to die suddenly, or (for a doctor) to attempt resuscitation on a patient

CODE STATUS: decision about what should be done in the event of sudden death; typically either full code (all measures should be taken to attempt to revive the patient) or DNAR (do not attempt resuscitation)

COPD: chronic obstructive pulmonary disease; lung diseases generally caused by long-term smoking, including chronic bronchitis and emphysema

CORONARY: having to do with the blood vessels to the heart

CPR: cardiopulmonary resuscitation

CRIXIVAN: common medication for HIV

CRYPTOCOCCUS: type of invasive fungal infection

CSF: cerebrospinal fluid; fluid encasing the brain and spinal cord, typically sampled via a lumbar puncture or "spinal tap," a hollow needle placed through the low back into the spinal column

CT SCAN: computed tomography scan; also called CAT (computed axial tomography); special form of X-ray that uses computer technology to create cross-sectional images ("slices") of the area being scanned

CVA: cerebrovascular accident; stroke

DECEREBRATE POSTURE: body posture indicating loss of function of the higher brain (cerebrum)

DETOX: detoxification program, aimed at eliminating physical dependence on alcohol or drugs (constrast to rehab, which addresses both physical and psychological addiction)

DIC: disseminated intravascular coagulation, disorder in which blood clots form in blood vessels throughout the body, paradoxically associated with abnormal bleeding as well; occurs in severe infections and other disorders; usually life threatening

DNAR: do not attempt resuscitation; decision not to attempt to restart the heart and lungs in the event of sudden death

DNR: DNAR (variant)

EMD: electromechanical dissociation; heart stoppage with normal electrical activity but no heart muscle response; also called PEA, pulseless electrical activity

ENCEPHALOPATHY: dysfunction of the brain

ENDOTRACHEAL TUBE: tube placed into the trachea (breathing tube) to allow artificial ventilation by a ventilator (breathing machine)

EPI: epinephrine (*see*)

EPINEPHRINE: adrenaline, a powerful body substance that is produced naturally but can also be given artificially to restart the heart and raise blood pressure, among other effects

ER: Emergency Room

ESOPHAGEAL: located in the esophagus (swallowing tube)

EXTUBATE: to remove an artificial breathing tube

FAMILIAL MEDITERRANEAN FEVER: a rare inherited disorder characterized by recurrent fevers and inflammation of the abdominal cavity

FIBRILLATION: irregular electrical and muscular activity (*see* atrial *and* ventricular)

FLUOROSCOPY: a type of real-time X-ray

FUNDOSCOPIC EXAM: examination of the back of the eye (fundus)

GASTROENTEROLOGIST: specialist in the gastrointestinal system, including stomach, intestines, liver, and pancreas

GI BLEED: gastrointestinal bleeding; blood in vomit or feces, from bleeding in the stomach or intestines

GRAM STAIN: a method of staining samples of tissue or bacteria to assist in microscopic identification

H. FLU: *hemophilus influenzae,* common bacteria causing pneumonia and other infections

HEMATOCRIT: red blood cell count; measurement of anemia (blood loss or failure to produce red blood cells)

HEME-ONC: abbreviation for hematology/oncology specialist or service

HEPATOCELLULAR CARCINOMA: liver cell cancer, a type particularly aggressive and difficult to treat

HEPATOMA: short for hepatocellular carcinoma

HOUSE STAFF: collective term for doctors in specialty training, including interns and residents

HYPERCOAGULABLE: excessive clotting of the blood

HYPERESTHESIA: abnormally strong sensation

ICU: Intensive Care Unit

IMMUNOSUPPRESSION: abnormal function of the immune system, as occurs in HIV/AIDS, blood cancers, and many severe chronic illnesses

INTERN: doctor in the first year of training after medical school; first-year resident

INTRAVASCULAR: within the veins and arteries

INTUBATE: to place a tube from the mouth into the trachea to allow artificial breathing by a breathing machine (ventilator)

IV: intravenous

JOHNNIE: hospital gown

LACTULOSE: medication given to reduce brain effects of liver disease

LIDOCAINE: medication given locally as an anesthetic (numbing medication) or intravenously to reduce abnormal heart rhythms

LYTIC: thrombolytic (*see*)

MEDIASTINUM: area of the chest between the lungs and the breastbone, including the heart, great vessels, lymph nodes, etc.

MENINGOCOCCUS: *Neisseria meningotides,* a bacteria that can cause infection of the brain, throat, and other areas

METASTASES: cancer cells that have migrated from their original location and created growths elsewhere in the body

METASTATIC: general term for having spread from an original location; generally refers to cancers but can also be used to describe infections

METS: short for metastases (*see*)

MILIARY: form of tuberculosis with tiny pockets of infection in multiple areas of the body

MRI: magnetic resonance imaging; scan that uses large magnets to create cross-sectional images of the areas being scanned

NASOGASTRIC TUBE (NG): tube placed through the nose down the esophagus into the stomach

NEB: short for nebulizer (*see*)

NEBULIZER (NEB): aerosolized medication; commonly albuterol (*see*)

NEPHROLOGIST: kidney specialist

NEPHROTOXIN: medication with the side effect of damage to the kidney

NEURO: abbreviation for neurology or neurologist

NG: nasogastric tube (*see*)

NOCARDIA: type of invasive fungal infection

NODULORETICULAR: pattern of tiny spots with lacy connections seen on an X-ray

NONSTEROIDAL ANTI-INFLAMMATORY DRUG (NSAID OR NONSTEROIDAL): one of a group of medications that reduce pain and inflammation, including ibuprofen (Advil or Motrin), naproxen (Aleve), and others

NSAID: nonsteroidal anti-inflammatory medication (*see*)

OCTREOTIDE: medication used to constrict the blood vessels of the esophagus and reduce bleeding from esophageal varices

OSHA: Occupational Health and Safety Administration; government agency that oversees safety measures in health care and elsewhere

OR: Operating Room

OXYCODONE: common narcotic pain medication

PANCREAS: an organ in the upper abdomen that makes digestive enzymes as well as insulin, and other hormones to control blood sugar

PANCREATITIS: inflammation or infection of the pancreas, often a severe and life-threatening disease

PAPILLEDEMA: swelling of the back of the eye, indicating dangerous elevation of pressure in the head from infection, swelling, or bleeding

PARACENTESIS: removal of fluid from the abdominal cavity, typically done when there is ascites (excessive fluid)

PEA: pulseless electrical activity; heart stoppage with normal electrical activity but no heart muscle response

PHEOCHROMOCYTOMA: a rare type of tumor typically arising from the adrenal glands, that secretes adrenaline and related hormones, causing sweating, palpitations, and extreme high blood pressure

PNEUMOCOCCUS: *streptococcus pneumoniae,* a bacterium that can cause pneumonia and other infections

PPD: purified protein derivative, a skin test for tuberculosis exposure

PREROUNDING: work done by an intern to gather information about patients before rounds

PROPHYLAXIS: measure taken to prevent development of disease

PULMONOLOGIST: lung specialist

PULMONARY EMBOLUS (PE): blood clot in the lungs (often life threatening)

PUPILLARY: having to do with the pupils of the eye

RESIDENT: doctor in training for a specialty; typically used to refer to those who have completed their first year in training (internship)

RHEUMATOLOGIST: joint specialist

ROUNDS: general term for the review of patients in a variety of settings; most often used to refer to a care team of students, interns, residents, and an attending walking around the hospital in the morning seeing and discussing each of the team's patients

SALSALATE: medication used to reduce inflammation in the intestines

SARCOIDOSIS: a poorly understood disease that causes inflammation and damage to multiple areas of the body including the lungs and heart

SCLERAE: whites of the eyes

SCLERODERMA: an autoimmune disease that causes scarring of the blood vessels and connective tissue

SIGN-OUT: information given about a patient to a doctor who will be covering their care over a night or weekend when their usual doctor is absent

SINUS TACHYCARDIA (SINUS TACH): rapid heart rate originating from the heart's normal pacemaker (the sinus node)

SPINAL TAP: removal of fluid from around the spinal cord; *see* CSF

STATUS EPILEPTICUS: continuous or prolonged seizure; often life threatening

SWAN-GANZ CATHETER (SWAN): catheter running from a vein through the heart into the lungs, to allow continuous monitoring of pressure and flow in multiple areas of the heart and lungs

TACHYCARDIA: rapid heart rate

THROMBOLYTIC: medication given to dissolve blood clots

TTP: thrombophilic thrombocytopenic purpura, a disorder that affects the kidneys, the platelets, and the red blood cells, and leads to mental confusion, rashes, blood clots, and excessive bleeding

TOX SCREEN: blood and/or urine test for multiple drugs and medications

TRICHOMONAS: common sexually transmitted infection

TUBE: short for "intubate" (*see*) or "endotracheal tube" (*see*)

TUBED: short for "inbated"

ULTRASOUND: test using sound waves to create an internal image of a part of the body

VARICES: enlarged veins; typically used to refer to the engorged veins in the esophagus seen in liver disease, which can cause life-threatening bleeding

VDRL: blood test for syphilis

VENTILATOR (VENT): artificial breathing machine

VENTRICULAR FIBRILLATION (V-FIB): heart stoppage caused by erratic contraction of the ventricles (large chambers) of the heart

XIPHOID: small triangular bone at the bottom of the sternum (breastbone)